The Complete
Massage
Tutor

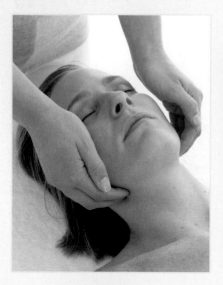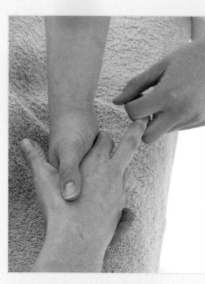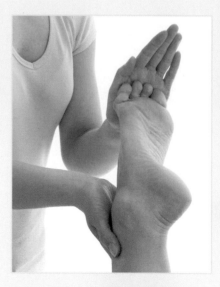
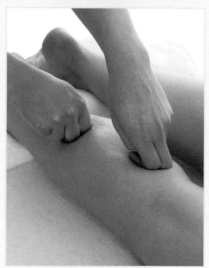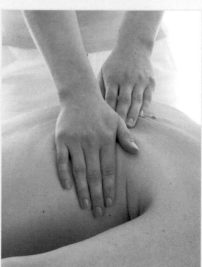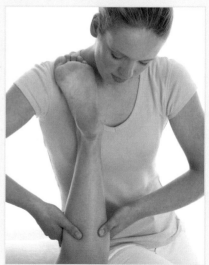
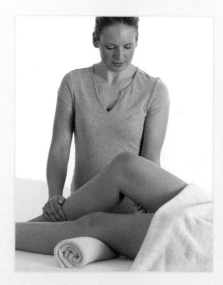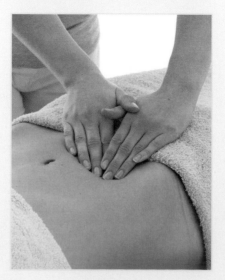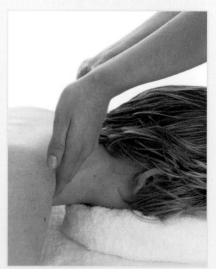

The Complete
Massage Tutor

*A structured course to achieve
professional expertise*

Wendy Kavanagh

An Hachette UK Company
www.hachette.co.uk

First published in Great Britain in 2010 by Gaia,
a division of Octopus Publishing Group Ltd
2–4 Heron Quays, London E14 4JP
www.octopusbooks.co.uk
www.octopusbooksusa.com

Distributed in the U.S. and Canada by Octopus
Books USA:
c/o Hachette Book Group USA
237 Park Avenue
New York NY 10017

Paperback ISBN: 978-1-856-75303-6
Hardback ISBN: 978-1-856-75323-4

A CIP catalogue record for this book is
available from the British Library

Printed and bound in China

10 9 8 7 6 5 4 3 2 1

All reasonable care has been taken in the
preparation of this book, but the information it
contains is not meant to take the place of medical
care under the direct supervision of a doctor.
Before making any changes in your health regime,
always consult a doctor. While all the therapies
detailed in this book are completely safe if done
correctly, you must seek professional advice if
you are in any doubt about any medical condition.
Any application of the ideas and information
contained in this book is at the reader's sole
discretion and risk.

Contents

Introduction

In recent years massage therapy has continued to evolve and with it, standards of education and training have risen. In many countries the profession is regulated either voluntarily or statutorily and this has required training to be formalized.

To be accepted as part of an integrated health system, a massage therapist will need to have a basic medical knowledge of the human body and its functions and to work ethically. Once considered a luxury, massage is becoming very much mainstream as a tool to combat the stresses of modern lifestyle. It is increasingly being used within or alongside orthodox medicine for its non-intrusive benefits.

Massage may be sought after for theraputic or relaxation purposes and there are a wide range of techniques to meet distinct needs. Most therapists specialize in several modalities, undertaking separate training for each and enabling them to integrate their body work and offer a treatment to suit the client's requirements and physical condition.

Massage is often referred to as a 'healing art', but uniquely it is both an art and a science, the art of the therapist in applying the strokes and the science of how these strokes promote well-being and the body's natural healing process. This book aims to combine the historical origins of massage with the requirements of a modern-day health care professional.

How to use this book

This book is aimed at those with an interest in starting a career in massage therapy. It can be used alongside course textbooks as an overview of some of the main elements that massage training establishments are required to teach.

In a user-friendly way, the text covers both the science of anatomy and physiology and the practical application of massage strokes. The book then moves on from these basic elements to what happens once training is complete, from setting up a massage practice to the common ailments that may present themselves.

The skill of a massage therapist comes from the way massage strokes are applied to acheive optimum benefit, in an holistic environment. The text will help understand the importance of preparation and need for communication and awareness.

The photography accompanying the step-by-step techniques make the book a user-friendly and enjoyable study guide.

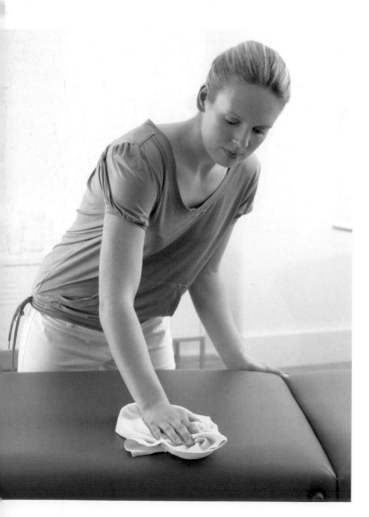

Preparation A good massage therapist will not only have the skills of massage, but will also have the knowledge to create a safe and holistic environment in which to practise.

Massage The book will take you through the basic strokes to a whole massage sequence, specialized massage routines and massage for common ailments.

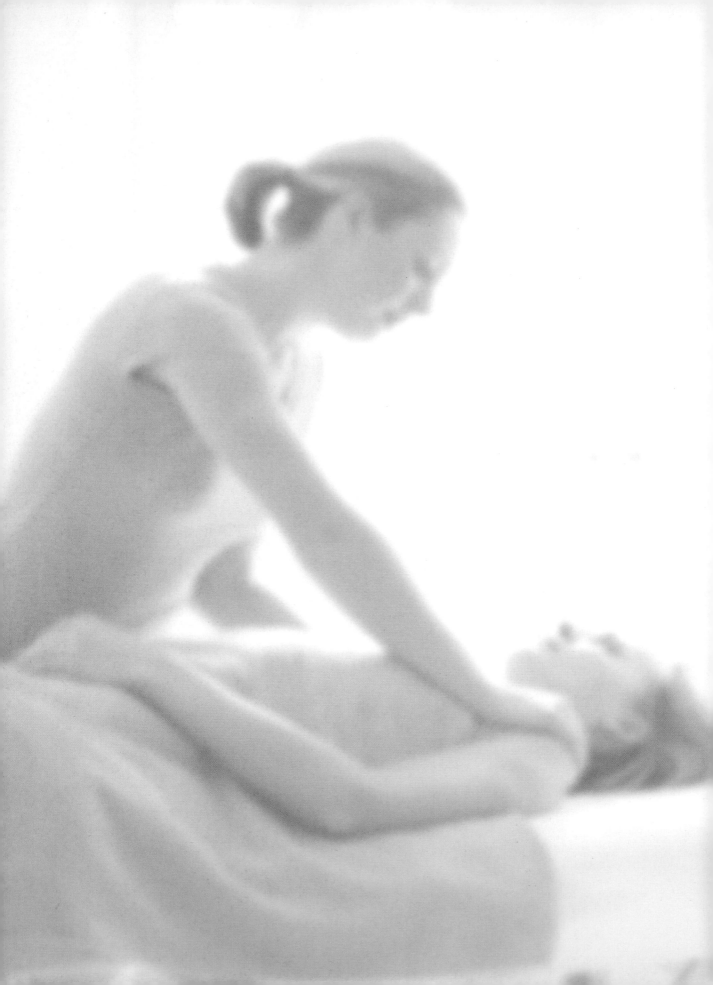

The origins of massage

Whether defined in clinical terms as 'the systematic and scientific manipulation of the soft tissue' or in more down-to-earth terms as 'the rubbing or kneading of parts of the body', massage is considered by many people to be a necessary catalyst in restoring and maintaining balance to physical, emotional and spiritual well-being. Massage in a variety of forms has been practised around the world for thousands of years, and its benefits are well documented.

The history of massage

It is important for any massage student or therapist to understand the origins and the development of the profession they have chosen and its legacy. A broad understanding of massage theory and a sense of identity makes for a well-informed and inspired practitioner.

The origin of the word 'massage' is unclear. Some say it comes from the Greek word *masso* or *massein*, 'to knead', which is descriptive of a type of technique that forms part of massage as practised today. Others trace the word to the arabic verb *mass* 'to touch', which may then have evolved into the French word *masser*. The term 'therapeutic' comes from the Greek, *therapeutikos* relating to the effect of a medical treatment. In the USA before the 19th century the term 'frictio', from the Latin for rubbing or friction, was used for massage, whereas in India it was known as 'shampooing'.

With Greek, Arabic, Roman, Indian, Chinese and Japanese origins, the earliest recorded references to massage occurred around 2,500 BC and prehistorically, cave paintings in Europe dated 15,000 BC depict what could be the practice of healing touch.

The chronology of massage can be divided into five distinct periods: Ancient World, Middle Ages to Renaissance, 19th century, modern age and the future:

COOK'S TREATMENT ON TAHITI

Captain Cook suffered badly with sciatica and rheumatism. On landing in Tahiti, a local native chief offered to help relieve the conditions by engaging the help of the female practitioners in the village. It is documented in Cook's diaries that he had 12 women pummelling his body while he was spread out on mats on the ground. The women used their hands, fists, elbows, knees and feet to work on all his muscles and joints. He was amazed that afterwards his pain was relieved, and he continued to receive 'treatments' during his stay, which resulted in the condition being alleviated.

The Ancient World

In the 25th century BC a medical text known as *Nei Ching* contains the earliest Chinese reference to the knowledge of massage, a style known as 'amma' or 'amna'. It describes techniques and their uses which went on to become well established. By the time of the T'ang dynasty, formal institutions were in place, including a Department of Massage.

Extensive visual evidence has been found in Egypt from the 24th century BC, including wall paintings depicting massage and reflexology decorating the tomb of Ankhmahor (the physician's tomb) in Saqqara. Around the same time, Persian and Japanese references to the benefits and usefulness of massage began to appear.

References to massage in the form of rubbing and shampooing appear in the Indian texts on the *Ayurveda* or 'Code of Life' from the 19th century BC, suggesting it as a means of helping the body to heal itself. *Samvahan* translated as 'hand rubbing', *makch* meaning 'to strike' or 'to press' and *mordan* to rub are mentioned in the Sanskrit literature.

Between the 5th and 1st centuries BC, massage entered a golden age, with a revolution in medical and physical therapies in Greece and Rome. The philosophy and practice of Hippocrates has been documented more than any other. He claimed that muscle tone and joint function could be improved by 'rubbing' and that strokes should be carried out in a direction towards the heart as is advocated today. In his treatise *On Joints*, published in about 400 BC, Hippocrates says 'the physician must be skilled in many things and particularly friction'.

Another advocate of massage was Galen of Pergamon, who combined Greek anatomy and

Massage in India This painting from 1825 shows a male attendant performing a leg massage. Traditionally, this would have been been done by personal servants.

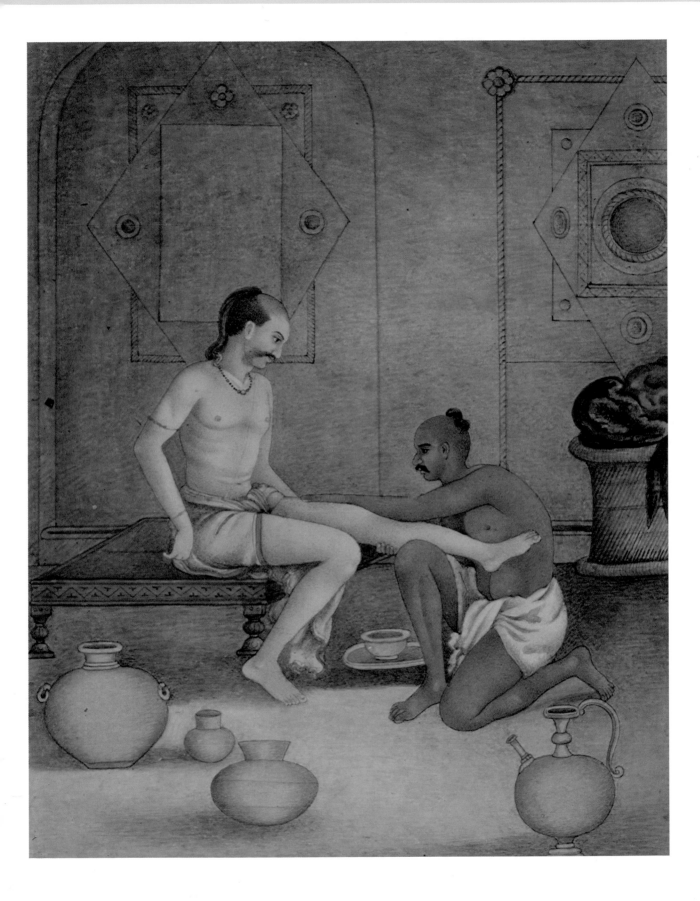

medicine in a system that survived the Middle Ages and dominated medicine for centuries.

Other references in this period came from Homer's *Odyssey*, in which he describes how exhausted war heroes were treated to oil rubdowns for restorative purposes. Elsewhere, regular massages were administered to gladiators to ease muscle fatigue and pain and Julius Caesar was 'pinched' all over daily as a treatment for neuralgia.

From the Middle Ages to the Renaissance

With the fall of the Roman Empire and the advent of the Christian era, massage as a treatment went into a period of decline. Although it survived in its healing art form, being used by folk healers and midwives, massage lost favour with the establishment. Religion focused on the soul and not the body – even the Olympic Games came to an end – and it was considered inappropriate to include massage in medical literature.

Of course there were some exceptions to the decline: Rhazes, a Persian physician, discussed massage in a major work about Greek, Roman and Arabic medical practices, and another important work at this time was the *Avicenna*, the canon of Arab philosopher and physician Ali Abu Ibn Szinna. This contained thoughts on the health-promoting properties of massage, and stated that combined with hydrotherapy it could help to disperse muscle by-products that are not expelled by exercise.

After its suppression in the Middle Ages, massage made a great comeback in the 16th century. The Renaissance was an exciting period and many prominent physicians incorporated bodywork into their approaches to treatment, including the eminent physician Ambrose Pare, medical advisor to four French kings, who classified the type of massage movements he employed. Mary Queen of Scots was also restored to health after a grave illness through the application of massage techniques by her doctor.

There are numerous documentations from the 17th and 18th centuries, during which the medical profession regained its prestige and massage took a great leap forward worldwide. Great strides in research were made by the Italian physiologist Giovanni Alfonso Borelli, who analyzed muscle contraction, and the English physician William Harvey, who worked on blood flow.

The 19th century

It was early in the 19th century that perhaps the most documented development in massage took place. A Swedish gymnast, Per Henrik Ling, combined his knowledge of philosophy and gymnastics with bodywork techniques that he had acquired during his travels to China. The combination of five basic strokes was known as 'the Swedish Movement' or 'Swedish massage' as we call it today and it is still practised in much the same way. These five strokes have become the 'mother' strokes of massage and most Western techniques use them as their base.

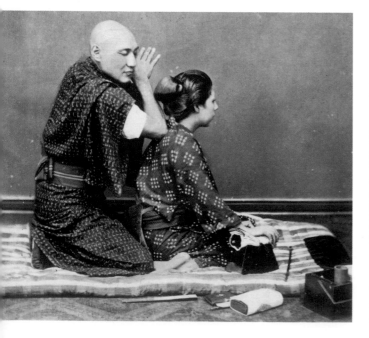

PROFESSIONAL BODIES

The world's first professional association for massage practitioners was formed by five female nurses in the UK in 1894. It was called the Society of Trained Masseuses and was set up to raise the standard and reputation of massage. Britain then had a system in place of 'health visitors', which offered health services to poorer members of the community. Part of their training was massage and also included some instruction in medical gymnastics.

Late 19th century massage A Japanese masseur works on his client, using his elbows to relieve tension in his client's back.

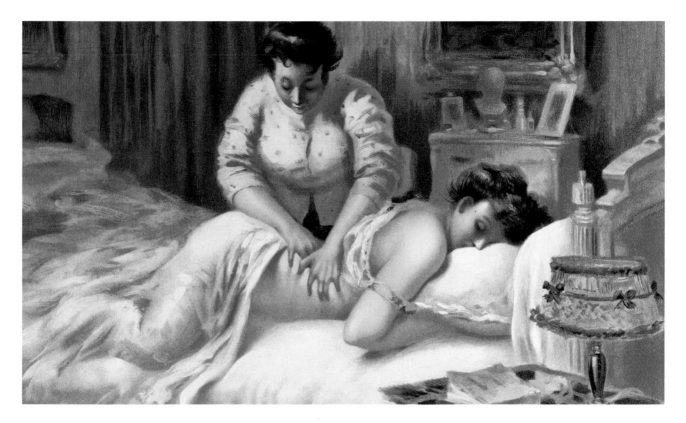

French massage This colour lithograph by Albert Guillaume shows a luxurious massage session in France during the 19th century.

The use of Swedish massage spread rapidly; the first college with massage on the curriculum was established in 1813. Then in 1850 the first book in English on the Swedish Movement was written by Dr Mathias Roth. Many medical physicians trained in massage, convinced of its usefulness alongside traditional procedures. This development led to an increase of publications from such writers as Mezger, Taylor, Graham, Nissen and Dr John Harvey Kellogg, whose 1895 book *The Art of Massage* included research into the effects of massage that were consistent with writings over the following 50 years.

The modern age

During the First World War, the Military Massage Service was set up to help treat the war wounded, as documented by James Mennell in his book *Physical Treatment by Movement, Manipulation and Massage*. The service was later revived in 1939. In civilian life, the Society of Trained Masseuses was set up in Britain in 1894 and then merged with the Chartered Society of Massage and Medical Gymnastics, to form a body with over 12,000 members.

But the biggest turnaround in the modern age was generated in the 1960s and 1970s from the Esalen Centre in California, USA, where massage was used intuitively and considered to be a powerful means to promote personal growth. As we now know, this holistic way of connecting mind, body and spirit brings us back full circle to how it began over three thousand years ago.

The future

So where do we stand in the 21st century? Massage has become part of mainstream complementary therapy and integrated medicine. Soft-tissue massage therapy is even being used in programmes acclimatizing astronauts to Earth's gravity on their return from space. It is part of everyday life and regularly discussed throughout the media. Research institutes are continuing to collate information on evidence-based effects and benefits. Practitioners are applying a broader range of techniques with specialisms and there is more emphasis on training, ethics and boundaries.

Massage has survived since prehistoric times; there have been golden ages when its popularity was unquestioned and periods when it fell into disrepute and was pushed underground. Across the globe, massage is in the process of being formalized and regulated, and there is no doubt that its future is very promising.

Introduction to massage therapy

The start of a career in massage therapy often begins with receiving treatments and experiencing their benefits, or a friend or colleague commenting that 'you have healing hands'. Many people change their working lives to follow this very satisfying and fulfilling profession, but what are the qualities required to become a massage therapist?

The first consideration is to the clients; they must be provided with a competent, safe treatment that is administered within a professional framework. To achieve this requires formal training in technical skills, the underpinning knowledge and, importantly, the handling of the client/therapist relationship within a code of ethics.

Besides an aptitude for working with his or her hands, a therapist needs to have good communication skills, both oral and written, so that clients are put at ease and client records prepared and maintained. It is most important that the therapist projects a professional image and works within set boundaries, including client confidentiality, trustworthiness and the ability to maintain a professional distance and detachment.

Intuitive technique Methods can be studied and applied, but a good therapist will also develop a connection and empathy with their clients.

A competent therapist recognizes the limits of their work. Massage therapists do not work diagnostically and cannot provide other services or therapies that they are not trained in; however, they should be able to refer a client elsewhere if appropriate. This may feel restrictive at times but there are other ways to 'add value' to the treatment by encouraging clients to pursue a healthy lifestyle and suggest preventive measures, including self-care massage.

Finally, good listening skills are essential; an important part of the work is daily contact on a very personal level with a wide variety of people, which requires a high level of understanding and empathy.

Once the basic sequence of strokes have been absorbed, a massage therapist can start to work intuitively, readily sensing sources of tension or imbalance and adapting the routine to the client's needs. A natural rhythmical and continual flow of strokes is the key to achieving good massage technique.

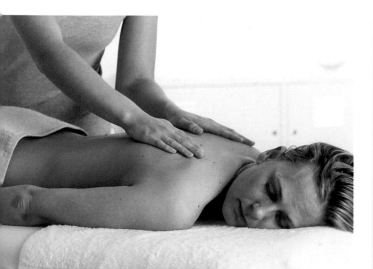

THE HEALTH OF THE THERAPIST

To achieve a comfortable and beneficial massage treatment, there needs to be a two-way flow between the giver and receiver. This interaction of touch and response means that the therapist has to prepare to give, while the client must allow them to do so in order for it to be effective. With this in mind it is not useful to practise massage if you are feeling stressed or tense, or you are not in full health, as energy levels will be depleted. A client will sense if a therapist is not focused and that care and sensitivity is not present; this may result in them going elsewhere for future treatments.

Massage for today

Increasingly, our modern way of life with its social pressures brings with it physical and emotional stresses. There is a constant drive towards high levels of achievement that are often unrealistic, while new technology means that divisions between work and personal time have become blurred and unbalanced. Diet, exercise and health are often neglected while trying to 'keep all the balls in the air'.

Alongside this self-inflicted stress there are other factors outside of our control that may be detremental to our well-being. These include pollution, emissions and chemicals in food products, to name a few. Stress-related illnesses such as irritable bowel syndrome, back pain, repetitive strain injury and ME have become increasingly common, If they are not addressed, these chronic conditions, many of which are preventable, if not curable, can seriously undermine a person's quality of life, as well as their work and participation in society.

The body's natural resilience to stress can easily become overwhelmed, leading to increased muscle tension, high blood pressure and over-stimulation, releasing cholesterol into the circulatory system. Massage therapy can play an important preventative role in combating these effects. It is one of the most effective ways to relax and unwind, whether applied in the form of simple self-massage or by visiting a qualified therapist on a regular basis. Devoting time to oneself during the massage and emptying the mind of all the pressures of the day is beneficial in itself.

Many companies recognize the pressures that today's workloads place on their employees and as part of their health in the workplace policies, offer the services of an on-site massage therapist. Using a specially designed chair or desk attachment, dynamic massage treatments can be given through the clothes in 20-minute sessions to relax and re-energize staff and address any work-related conditions that may occur.

In many traditional cultures regular massage is accepted as part of daily life for all ages. In recent years the West has seen treatments becoming more accessible as massage practice has spread from the world of sport into wider society.

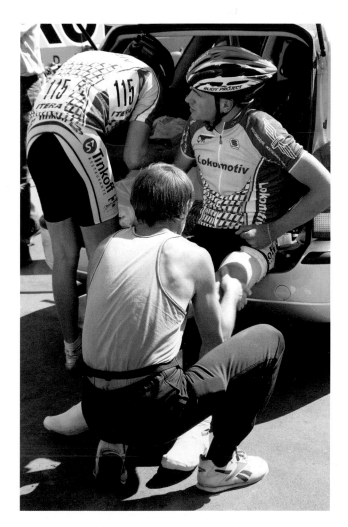

Sports massage Massage has been a useful tool in treating athletes and sportspeople for many years, and has now become a much more common therapy.

Who can benefit from massage?

There are no limits to who can benefit from massage therapy. It can be practised from the cradle to the grave and is one of the safest, least intrusive therapies. It is one of the most popular and widely used complementary therapies due to its versatility and compatability with other therapies.

Although training establishments teach massage techniques that can be applied to babies, children, adults and the elderly, the weak, healthy and terminally ill, there are a few conditions in which massage is contraindicated and it is important to be aware of these; they are described in Chapter 4.

Massage is regularly used alongside other therapies and in association with amateur and professional sports, palliative care, mental health, rehabilitation, anger management, the workplace, and also in clinics, spas and retreats. On a physical level, massage encourages the body's self-healing process by mechanically assisting the main physiological systems.

The benefits of massage can be broadly categorized into physical, emotional, psychological and energetic.

Physical

The physical conditions helped by massage include:

- **Muscular and skeletal conditions**: Massage benefits these through improved circulation of blood and stimulation of overlying muscles. It helps maintain muscles in the best possible state of nutrition, flexibility and vitality so that they can function well after recovery from trauma, disease or excessive exercise. Research shows that massage can also cause relaxation of voluntary muscles. It may also lessen the fibrosis that develops in immobilized, injured or denervated muscle. Deep-tissue massage reduces the formation of scar tissue and improves connective tissue healing. In the case of fractures, the promotion of blood flow to the new network of blood vessels that forms at the break site encourages healing.
- **Postural conditions**: When muscles and joints are free from tension, a wider range of movement is possible. This in turn results in better posture.
- **Circulatory conditions**: Improved blood circulation assisted by deep massage strokes helps to reduce

blood pressure, aid the expulsion of metabolic waste and increase blood cell count. The promotion of lymph flow strengthens the immune system and reduces build up of fluid.
- **Respiratory conditions**: By strengthening and relaxing the respiratory muscles, massage improves pulmonary function, which can reduce the severity of asthma attacks and slow down breathing.
- **Digestive conditions**: Abdominal massage promotes the production of digestive secretions and aids the absorption of food. The improvement in blood and lymph circulation creates a demand for an increased supply of nutrients, bringing about improvement in appetite.
- **Skin conditions**: Unless contraindicated (see Chapter 4), skin conditions, tone and texture may be improved by massage, as is the healing of any abrasions.
- **Pain relief**: Better circulation can relieve local and referred pain. The release of endorphins and other pain-reducing neurochemicals stimulated by massage interrupts the pain cycle, bringing short-term relief.

EMOTIONAL RELEASE

Sometimes massage treatments are used subconsciously to satisfy the emotional needs that nurturing touch fulfils, those of acceptance, care and attention. This can result in the release of emotion during treatment; the client may spontaneously laugh, sigh or cry. In very rare cases clients show anger as they let down their defences in the safety experienced with their therapist.

Emotional

The relaxation response evoked by massage affects the nervous system and reduces stress and anxiety, both in the receiver and giver of massage. Stress hormones and cortisol levels are reduced and nerves soothed. This relaxation can also improve sleep patterns for those with insomnia.

Changes of a chemical and physiological nature from negative to positive and the release of endorphins stimulated by massage reduce feelings of depression.

Psychological

Clients receiving regular massage become more body-aware. This becomes a journey of self discovery as the client learns how it feels to be relaxed and in tune with their well-being. Clients also develop an increased awareness of what is happening in different parts of their bodies. This all helps the process of taking responsibility for one's own health and happiness.

For those who have been sensitive or averse to touch because of negative associations, massage plays an important role in reducing these feelings and making touch a more comfortable experience.

Poor body image and low self-esteem have been known to decrease after massage treatment, as individuals become more comfortable and knowledgeable about their bodies.

Energy levels

With increased feelings of well-being, many clients experience a sense of renewed energy. This can be emotional or the result of better physical mobility. Sports massage is a good example of the use of massage to enhance performance. Professional athletes claim that pre-event treatment plans can increase efficiency by up to 20 per cent.

By relaxing the body and mind and removing stress with massage, an increase in mental alertness may occur that can help with academic studies. On a more spiritual level, as taught in Eastern therapies, the body has energy centres called chakras and energy channels known as ki or qi. It is believed that certain massage techniques stimulate these centres and promote the flow of ki, removing any 'blockages' or negative energy in order to re-energize the body. Chapters 7 and 8 look at specialized massage in more depth.

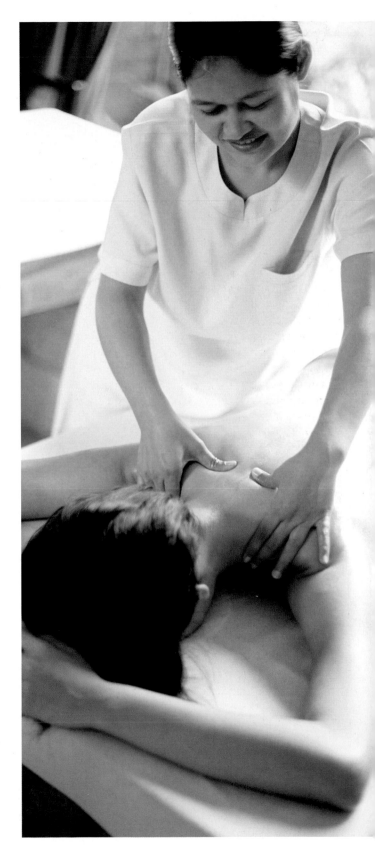

Relaxing the body Massage can be highly beneficial in relieving muscular and skeletal conditions and promoting relaxation in muscles that carry high levels of tension.

Clinical evidence and research

Research is a fundamental aspect of conventional medicine and health care, as it supports the theory and helps to identify treatments that offer the most benefit. The key to the acceptance of massage and other complementary therapies within the mainstream health care system is to provide evidence that evaluates the benefits and effects through a sizeable body of research.

For the average massage therapist, research may seem difficult and hard to understand, but being able to locate and read research gives you a valuable tool in offering the best treatment possible to your client. It keeps you abreast of current trends and the latest developments, and may help in your treatment planning.

There are numerous ways to locate research studies or journal articles, the most accessible of these being computerized databases that are publicly available. The most widely used database in medicine at present is the one maintained by the National Library of Medicine in Bethesda, Maryland, known as MEDLINE, which has a section that can be accessed on line entitled PubMed. Although most of the clinical research on massage is currently being carried out in the USA, many countries are now building their own complementary medicine research databases that can be subscribed to. Some journals are also published on-line and contain relevant research articles.

DR TIFFANY FIELD

Clinical research into massage therapy originated with the work of Dr Field who massaged her premature baby. She found that this produced a calming effect and, as a professor of paediatrics and psychiatry, decided to study prematurity and massage. Her research work in 1982 was conducted before massage was accepted as a popular treatment by doctors and the general public. She is now recognized as the foremost expert in touch research.

Research studies

Research papers follow a specific format, starting with a title and a list of authors; then an abstract, which is a summary of main points covering the context, purpose or objective of the research; then a simple description of the methodology employed and how it was carried out; and finally the results and the author's conclusions and references used. References to such papers will list the authors, title, name of publication, date of publication and page numbers.

There are two broad categories of clinical studies: observational and experimental. Observational studies look at a natural course of events and the outcomes in order to collate data and draw conclusions, whereas experimental studies require the implementation of a treatment programme by the researcher.

Massage therapists conducting research in their own practices frequently use the experimental 'before-and-after' study as a useful and practical way of measuring effects and benefits, though the more formal clinical trial, sometimes called a randomized controlled trial (RCT), is the most accepted evidence by conventional medical practitioners.

Despite the vast amount of material from around the world, and establishments such as the Touch Research Institute at the University of Miami, there still needs to be more formal research into massage if we are to bridge the gap between conventional and complementary practices.

Learning to understand research during our training will improve our ability to communicate with other health professionals in a common language, which in turn may lead to a better understanding and appreciation of our skills.

When we discuss research and massage, one of the most important developments in the last 15 years has

Personal research Therapists can conduct their own research into the efects and benefits of massage on their clients using the 'before and after' research method.

been the establishment of the Touch Research Institute, founded as a result of the pioneering work of Dr Tiffany Field, professor of paediatrics, psychology and psychiatry at the University of Miami, Florida. Dr Field started with a research project into the effects of massage on premature babies, taking 40 subjects and applying massage to one half of the group over a ten-day period, three times a day for 15-minutes. The outcome of the research was that the massaged babies gained 47 per cent more weight than those who did not receive massage. Other benefits confirmed were that the massaged babies were more alert, had better coordination skills, were more responsive and were able to leave hospital up to six days earlier than the unmassaged babies. The publication of Dr Field's research findings prompted Johnson & Johnson to fund the establishment of an Institute within the University of Miami devoted to the study of touch and its scientific and medical applications.

Since its inception in 1992, the Touch Research Institute has produced many studies on the effects of massage and touch at all stages of life, and has continued to work with premature babies and those born with addictions. Some of the more recent research programmes have been groundbreaking, dealing with areas that are sometimes considered contraindicated for massage. The papers are widely published and have been the inspiration for many other massage research programmes.

Baby massage Research shows that you are never too young to receive massage. Babies thrive on the power of touch, which promotes better sleeping and feeding patterns.

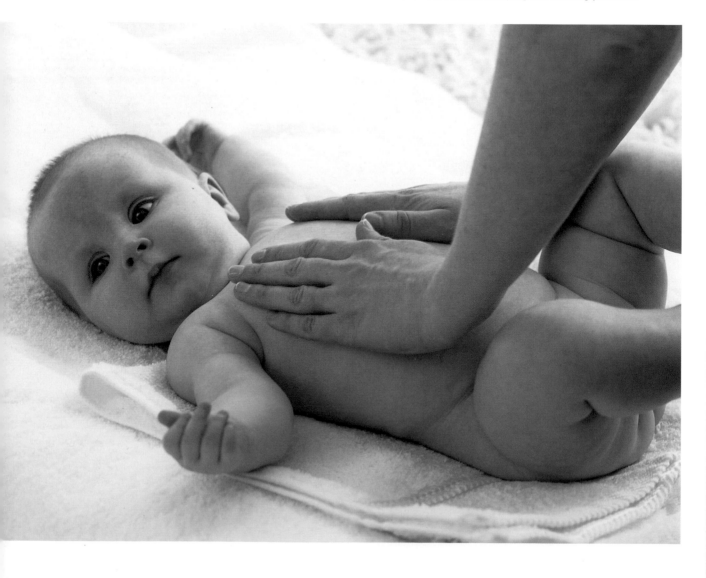

EXAMPLES OF RESEARCH

Tactile/kinesthetic stimulation effects on preterm neonates.

Preterm infants gained 47 per cent more weight, became more socially responsive, and were discharged six days earlier at a hospital cost savings of $10,000 per infant (or 4.7 billion dollars if the 470,000 preemies born each year were massaged). The underlying biological mechanism for weight gain in the massaged preterm newborns may be an increase in vagal tone and, in turn, an increase in insulin (food absorption hormone).
Field, T., Schanberg, S.M., Scafidi, F. et al. (1986). *Pediatrics* 77

Stable preterm infants gain more weight and spent less time sleeping and more time in the drowsy states following 5 days of massage therapy.

In a later study, preterm infants gained more weight following as few as five days of massage therapy.
Dieter, J., Field, T., Hernandez-Reif, M., Emory, E and Redzepi, M. (2003). *Journal of Pediatric Psychology* 28(6)

Massage stimulates growth in preterm infants: A replication.

Preterm infants receiving tactile/kinaesthetic stimulation over a 10-day period averaged 21 per cent greater weight gain per day and spent more time awake and active during sleep/wake behaviour observations than infants that were not massaged.
Scafidi, F., Field, T., Schanberg, S. et al. (1990). *Infant Behavior and Development* 13

Factors that predict which preterm infants benefit most from massage therapy.

Preterm infants received three daily 15-minute massages for 10 days. The massage therapy infants gained significantly more weight per day than did the control infants. For the massage therapy group, the pattern of greater caloric intake and more days in Intermediate care before the study period along with more obstetric complications differentiated the high from the low weight gainers, suggesting that the infants who had experienced more complications before the study benefited more from the massage therapy.
Scafidi, F., Field, T. and Schanberg, S. (1993). *Developmental and Behavioral Pediatrics* 14

Massage therapy facilitates weight gain in preterm infants.

Although the underlying mechanism for the relationship between massage therapy and weight gain has not yet been established, possibilities that have been explored in studies with both humans and rats include (a) increased protein synthesis, (b) increased vagal activity that releases food-absorption hormones like insulin and enhances gastric motility and (c) decreased cortisol levels leading to increased oxytocin.
Field, T. (2001). *Current Directions in Psychological Science* 10

Effects of tactile/kinesthetic stimulation on the clinical course and sleep/wake behavior of preterm neonates.

Preterm infants who were massaged before sleep fell asleep more quickly and slept more soundly with better sleep patterns. They showed improved weight gain compared with infants who were not massaged.
Scafidi, F., Field, T., Schanberg, S., Bauer, C., Vega-Lahr, N. and Garcia, R. (1986). *Infant Behavior and Development* 9

Sleep problems in infants decrease following massage therapy.

This study looked at the effectiveness of pre-bedtime massages for infants and toddlers with sleep onset problems. It was found that, compared with bedtime stories, massages produced fewer sleep delays and a shortened latency to sleep onset.
Field, T. and Hernandez-Reif, M. (2001). *Early Child Development and Care* 168

Massage of preterm newborns to improve growth and development.

Preterm infants who received massage therapy as newborns showed greater weight gain and more optimal cognitive and motor development eight months later.
Field, T., Scafidi, F. and Schanberg, S. (1987). *Pediatric Nursing* 13

Stable preterm infants gain more weight and sleep less after five days of massage therapy.

Healthy, low-risk preterm infants gained more weight and slept less with just five days of massage, in contrast to 10 days in previous studies. Results support the continued use of massage as a cost-effective therapy for medically stable preterm infants.
Dieter, J.N., Field, T., Hernandez-Reif, M., Emory, E.K. and Redzepi, M. (2003). *Journal of Pediatric Psychology* 28

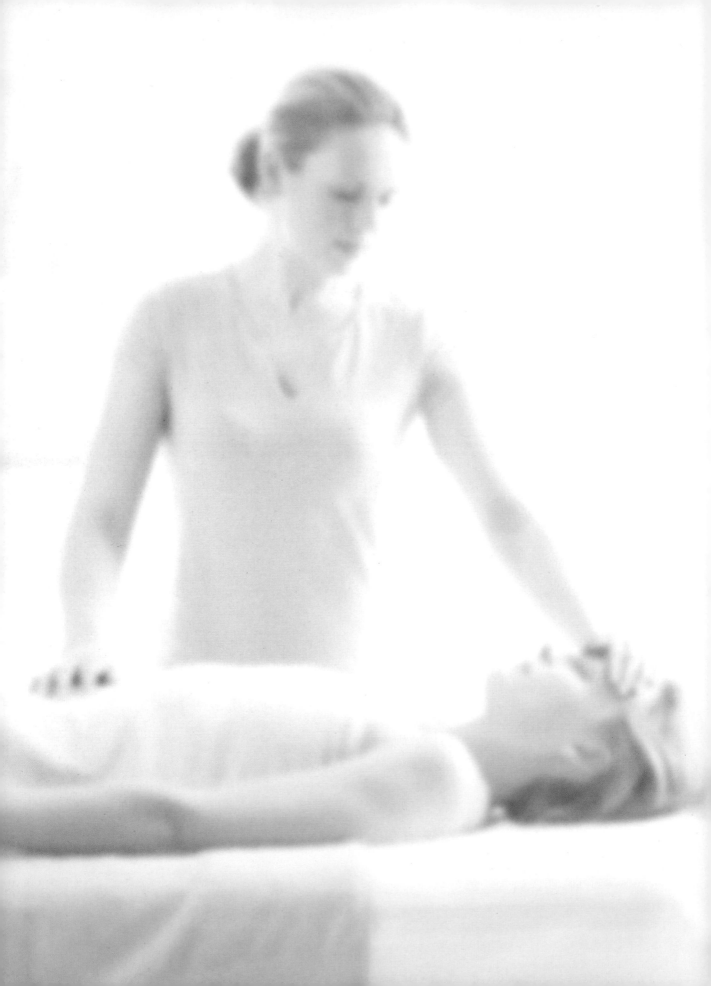

How does massage work?

The use of touch in a therapeutic form has been well documented over thousands of years. For centuries we have known that touch is good for us and that if received on a regular basis it results in a healthier and happier person, but what are the mechanics of the therapy and how does it work? In this chapter we introduce the physiology of touch and how the body's systems are affected by different forms of massage.

The language of touch

Human physiology is very complex and massage stimulates many of the processes underneath the skin, causing them to start up or enhancing their performance. Touch in this form sends messages to the brain and back in the form of chemical signals, which result in a combination of calming and stimulating effects.

One of the main hormones released in response to massage is oxytocin. Produced in the brain and released from nerve endings, oxytocin encourages relaxation and enhances a feeling of well-being. Another natural substance associated with massage and touch is endorphin, a neurotransmitter that acts as a natural mood enhancer and pain relief mechanism.

A major role of massage is to help maintain the homeostasis of the body. A formal definition of homeostasis is 'the maintenance of metabolic equilibrium within a body by compensating for disrupting changes'. Basically, this means that if the homeostasis of the body is maintained, the body's physiological systems are adapting internally to any changes in conditions externally.

A simple example of this is what happens within the body when the atmospheric temperature rises. The sensors in the skin detect the rise in temperature, messages are sent via the nervous system, which dilate the blood vessels near the skin, increasing blood flow so that the extra heat can be removed through conduction.

At the same time, sweat glands increase production of sweat, which then evaporates on the skin, cooling the body further in order for normal temperature levels to be maintained.

When massage is applied, the body responds in two ways, mechanically and reflexively. As connective tissue is manipulated, the pressure and range of motion results in mechanical responses, such as increased blood circulation, the relief of muscle tension and the reduction in scar tissue formation. In addition, reflexive responses occur when the nervous system is stimulated through the nerve endings in the skin. This in turn activates a reflex arc that can result in the promotion of general relaxation, decreased blood pressure and a reduction in respiratory rate.

The effects of massage are covered in greater detail in Chapter 3.

Communication via touch

Touch is the only sense that involves the whole of the body; the other four senses of smell, hearing, sight and taste reside in the head. The ability to feel touch is the first of the senses to develop in the human embryo, forming as early as the sixth week of pregnancy in the womb, and it serves an instinctive and primal need. For humans, and indeed for all animals, touch is vital for physical and mental health. Experiments with primates have proved that animals deprived of touch feel alone and isolated. This results in anxiousness, depression, poor development and a reduced sense of reality. In our society, solitary confinement is still considered a severe punishment.

The language of touch is what we use instinctively to express our feelings to others. It is the first means of communication available to us. As babies we use it is a way of exploring the world, obtaining food and bonding with our parents. Touch at this early stage in life equips

MASSAGE IN THE MOUNTAINS

A clear example of the power of touch is to be found in the training of blind and visually impaired massage therapists. In Nepal massage training has enabled a group of visually impaired people to become self-sufficient through offering massage to weary tourists who have been walking in the Himalayas. The quality of touch of these therapists is truly inspirational and a powerful communication tool.

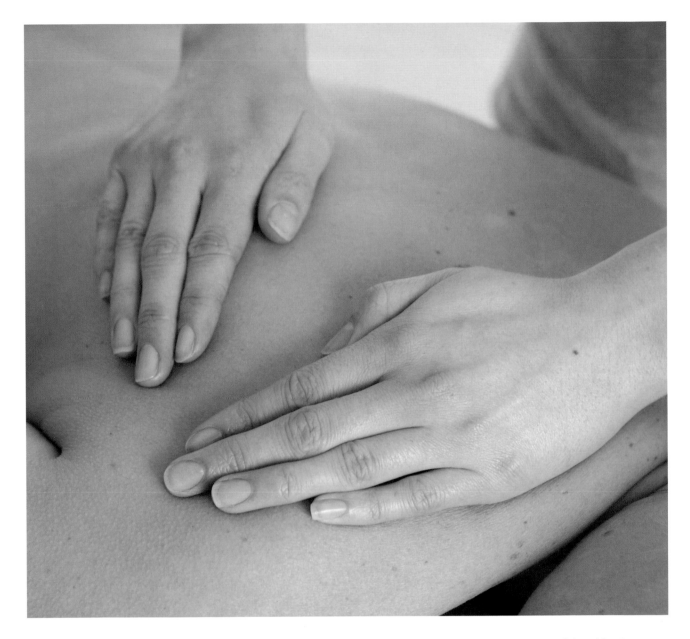

us later to build a healthy image of ourselves, when how often we are touched by others is related to esteem and self-value.

The skin, although in some senses a barrier to the outside world, also acts as a superficial nervous system. Each fingertip alone has about 700 touch receptors, allowing us to gather vast quantities of information through touch. For instance, it enables us to distinguish between deep or light pressure, high and low temperatures or different materials. An example of the power of this language is shown by the way people with impaired sight are able to visualize a person or object through touch.

Power of touch Touch is the most powerful tool for the massage therapist, relaying information about what lies under the skin through the touch receptors located on the fingertips.

Touch is also the natural response to pain and healing, a child will rub his or her bumps and bruises, adults rest their aching heads in their hands. Sympathy and reassurance is conveyed by holding or stroking. Recently dogs have been introduced into treatment for people following strokes or heart attacks as it has been found that stroking an animal is very therapeutic and promotes recovery.

The value of touch in the form of massage

Massage is the sharing of this language of touch, which is why the therapist benefits as well as the client; it is a two-way communication. In holistic massage this is particularly important and the body is treated as a whole with equal emphasis on communication and the physical conditions. The 'conversation' starts with the client's body telling you what needs addressing, the therapist responds with manipulation and the client's body reacts accordingly. With experience, each therapist will develop their own language of touch.

Clinicians and medical practitioners who use physical contact as an integral part of their work are very aware of the power of touch. Neuroscientists focusing on infant development have found that magnetic resonance imaging (MRI) scanners used in their work reveal how touch affects the maturing brain. They state that early experience by the child of secure attachment promoted by touch lays essential foundations for emotional and physiological stability in later years. Other researchers in the USA have demonstrated that this is not exclusive to childhood and that people, no matter what age or stage in life, remain open to changes in the body and brain as a result of touch. When a massage therapist places their hands on a client, an amazing amount of information is given out and received, and even the most mechanical bodywork can elicit an emotional response.

It is known from physiological studies that when touch is given in a caring, holistic manner it causes the release of the hormone oxytocin. Found at high levels in women while breast-feeding, oxytocin bonds mother and baby with feelings of love and security. In adults in general, this powerful hormone engenders feelings of well-being and nurturing.

The most uncomplicated language of touch is one we often forget – the warmth and human affection that is given and received through the skin in the form of a hug or a stroke.

Touch ability The ability to touch and feel is the first sense to develop in the human embryo and the first connection made between parent and child.

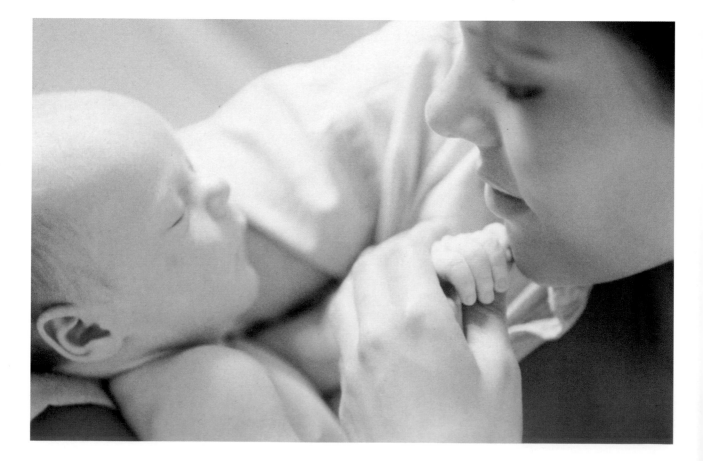

Overview of types of massage

There are well over 75 known different types of massage, generally divided into the Western physical based and the Eastern more spiritual based methods.

Although it has been around for centuries, the modern Western style of massage is largely based on Per Henrik Ling's 19th-century system of Swedish massage, incorporating the influences of modern sports and medicine. The emphasis is on the physical body and its conditions and using touch in the very physical sense.

Eastern techniques tend to have a more spiritual base, using theories of energy movement. These include mind, body and spirit and a persons' surroundings; the belief is that any change is not localized but affects the system as a whole. Touch is used to balance the whole system, not just the physical element.

It is useful for the student massage therapist to be aware of the variety of different types of massage practised and to have an underpinning knowledge of other body and complementary therapies.

As travel has become more affordable, people in Western Europe and America have been exposed to different treatments from around the world. Besides the Swedish-based massage systems there are three other increasingly popular therapies: Thai massage, Chinese massage (Tui-na) and Indian Head Massage. These are profiled in this chapter.

PER HENRIK LING

Ling's knowledge, accumulated on his travels to the Far East and Turkey, combined with a system of medical gymnastics called 'The Swedish Movement Cure' provided us with what is today known as Swedish Massage. There are still unanswered questions as to why the base techniques were interpreted by a Swedish man but have French terminology. One answer is that Ling's patron, King Charles XIV of Sweden was French, another that Ling was also the fencing master at the Swedish Royal Academy where all terminology was, and still is, in French.

Swedish massage

Originally developed by Swedish gymnast Per Henrik Ling (1776–1839), now considered the father of massage, this system arose from the combination of his knowledge of gymnastics and massage techniques acquired during his travels to China.

From 1813 to 1839 Ling taught in Sweden and his technique quickly caught on, being taught in 38 teaching institutes across Europe by 1851. Although massage was originally only part of the overall treatment, after his death it was taken out of context and practised alone as Swedish massage. This development has been credited to the Dutchman Johann Mezger (1817–1893), a follower of Ling, who organized the manipulations and introduced their French descriptions. As a physician he was more able to promote massage as a stand-alone treatment.

Mezger's combination using five basic strokes – effleurage, petrissage, friction, tapotement and vibration – and their variations, as well as two types of movement, is still practised in much the same way today. The strokes are applied hand to skin with the aid of a gliding agent in varying directions, pressures and speeds formatted in a series of movements or sequence, while the client is positioned on a massage table, chair or mat.

The second part of Ling's system, the movements, involve joint mobilization and stretching and can be applied before, during and after a massage treatment without the use of a lubricant. They are classified into two types: active and passive. Active movement is where the range of motion or stretching is performed by the client after demonstration from the therapist. Passive movement is performed by the therapist on the client in a relaxed state.

What does it treat?

Swedish massage is considered the 'grandparent' of Western massage techniques and can be used for relaxation purposes or to help in rehabilitation following injury. It also has many positive effects on general health, as documented in articles published by George Taylor, a doctor in New York in the late 1800s and the founder of

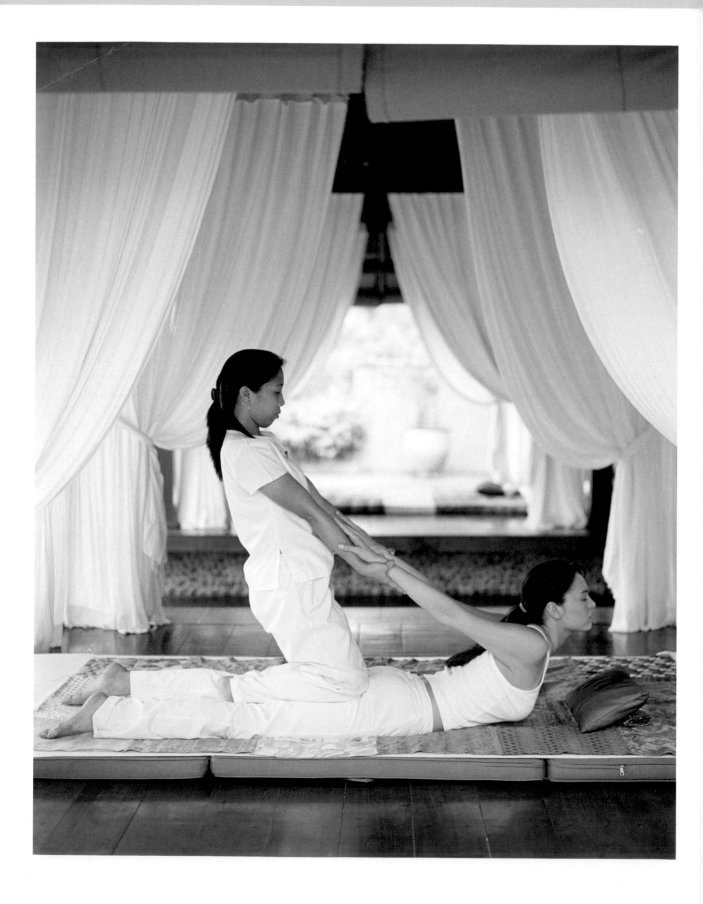

the first American school to teach Ling's methods. Modern-day Swedish-based massage is used in homes, clinics, surgeries and hospitals.

Chinese massage

An ancient form of Chinese bodywork, Tui Na (pronounced 'twee-nah') is integral to Traditional Chinese Medicine and translates as 'to push and grasp'. It was first mentioned in the *Nei Ching*, the medical encyclopaedia of the Yellow Emperor in the 25th century BC, which probably makes it the oldest form of bodywork still practised.

As with other Eastern types of bodywork, Chinese massage centres around the body's life energy or qi and is a hands-on therapy that takes place through loose comfortable clothing while the client is positioned on a floor mat, chair or massage table.

Soft tissue is manipulated using a unique 'rolling' action of the therapist's hands and forearms together with other techniques including kneading, chaffing and vibration. These massage movements, together with active and passive movements, are combined with applied pressure on specific pressure points located along meridians or pathways in order to free up the flow of energy.

The system recognizes a network of 12 paired meridians – one of each pair on the right side of the body and the other on the left. There are also two unpaired meridians that encircle the trunk and the head in the mid-line.

What does it treat?

Tui Na is useful in treating chronic pain and immobility problems, in particular those caused by musculoskeletal conditions and injuries of the upper body and back. Golfer's/tennis elbow, carpal tunnel syndrome and sciatica respond well to Chinese massage. As with Swedish massage, a wide range of conditions from migraines to irritable bowel syndrome can be alleviated, and in China, Tui Na is used for conditions that Western doctors would refer to osteopaths, chiropractors and physiotherapists.

Thai massage

Traditional Thai massage is known as Nuad Bo'Rarn in Thailand from the word *nuad* meaning 'massage' and

Thai massage This is a powerful technique where the therapist uses the whole of their body to apply pressure and some stretching.

ESALEN MASSAGE

One of the biggest developments in massage in recent years took place in the 1960s and 1970s when techniques were linked with a powerful means of promoting personal growth. Known for its long, integrating strokes, this truly holistic massage eminated from The Esalen Institute, California and combined the best from both Western and Eastern techniques translated into a unique massage form. People travel from around the world to be educated in this very effective healing art.

bo'rarn, which means 'traditional'. Massage techniques known as Thai massage are believed to have been introduced over 2,500 years ago by Buddhist monks who migrated from India to Thailand. Massage and medicine developed with the Buddhist teachings, being kept within the temple schools called 'wats'. Written massage and medical texts were treasured and kept in the King's palace until most were destroyed in 1767. In the mid-19th century the last remaining texts were inscribed on plaques preserved within the grounds of Wat Pho, in Bangkok, where they can still be viewed today. Many of the world's eminent Thai massage therapists learnt their craft at Wat Pho.

As in Chinese massage, the system works on the flow of energy through pathways. Thai massage is based on a belief that the body is composed of 72,000 channels or streams of qi energy, of which ten major lines or *sen sib* (translated as 'ten lines') are worked on by the therapist in a unique system that follows its own theory of flow and balance.

The technique is a blend of yoga and acupressure and uses point pressure, mobilization and rhythmic rocking applied through loose clothing without the use of a lubricant while the client is positioned on a floor mat. Each wat or temple teaches its own style. The Rural style involves closer contact between the therapist and client. Pressure is applied with thumbs, fingers, palms, forearms, elbows, knees and feet in four main positions – supine, side, prone and sitting. The Royal style is less intimate, with little stretching and the therapist applying pressure mostly with the thumb.

What does it treat?

Musculoskeletal pain and lack of mobility due to the shortening of muscles that occurs as a result of repetitive

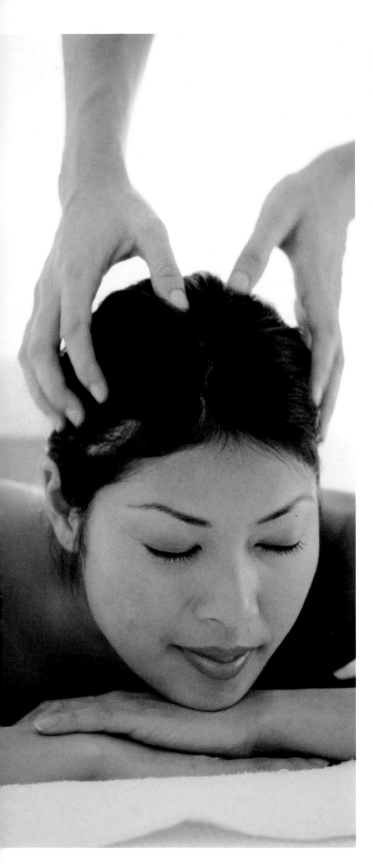

strain responds well to Thai massage, which is designed to stretch the muscles more than would be possible unaided. Regular massage stretches the muscle back to its normal resting length and before long tension and spasm disappear and mobility returns to normal.

Indian head massage

Head massage is just a small part of the vast Ayurvedic system of healing, that has been practised in India for over a thousand years. It is mentioned in the earliest Ayurvedic text, dating back to the 19th century BC, and has always played an important part of everyday Indian life, being performed by hairdressers and masseurs, as well as being used in rituals such as weddings and births. In the West it tends to be taken out of context and is often used as a standalone therapy.

Indian head massage was originally developed by women who used different oils according to the season and individualized techniques to keep their long hair strong, lustrous and in beautiful condition. Barbers practised many of the same skills with their male clients but included a *champiwas* – an invigorating scalp massage designed to stimulate and refresh.

In modern Western forms, therapists use a range of strokes from the Swedish system with additional compression movements over the neck, shoulder and scalp areas. In addition, they may also gently stimulate and stroke pressure points on the face. The treatment can be administered with or without oil while the client is in a seated position and fully clothed.

What does it treat?

Working on the head brings tremendous relaxation and is especially suited to relieving stress, tension, fatigue, insomnia, headaches, migraine and sinusitis. In addition, the oil used for massage serves as an excellent hair conditioner. The Ayurvedic text states that, when used in conjunction with herbs, spices and aromatic oils, massage had an important medical function and could not only 'strengthen muscles and firm skin', but also encourage the body's innate healing energy.

Indian head massage Techniques used in Indian head massage can be adapted and integrated into a table massage routine, with or without the use of oils.

Developing your own style

The first level of training in massage therapy is designed as a base to build on. Although the average client will be happy with your techniques when you are newly trained, the learning process does not end there.

You can compare training in massage with learning to drive a car: everyone takes the same training and test, but then their own style of driving evolves, some becoming advanced or HGV drivers, others remaining at the level they qualified. With hands-on experience and continuing professional development programmes, your style will develop and becomes personalized.

As you gain knowledge of other types of massage and bodywork, you can integrate these into the massage treatment where suitable. For example, if you have taken a course in trigger point therapy you can use this knowledge to help release muscle tension in situations where general massage is not so effective. This is often referred to as integrated bodywork.

Responding to client needs

Your style will change from client to client, depending on their needs and you will find your repertoire may range from a light, deeply relaxing treatment to deep tissue remedial work.

You will also need to adapt to individuals who have physical or emotional challenges. This could entail a simple use of repositioning in the case of a person who has spinal abnormalities or who is heavily pregnant, or the development of a specialized routine for paediatrics. In some cases the actual massage strokes you use will not change, instead it will be the length, pressure, speed and duration that will alter.

Take care of yourself

It is often underestimated how physical the work of a massage therapist is and how you need to take care of your own body. As you gain more experience and build up your massage practice, you will start to introduce further techniques that will reduce the pressure on your own body and increase the longevity of your career. A massage therapist should continually develop their style throughout their working life, often specializing in an area that interests them most. It is a true vocation.

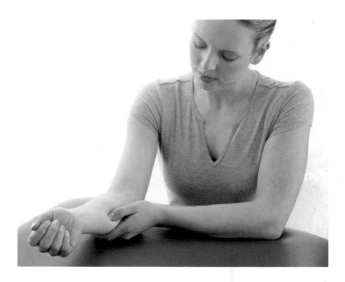

Self massage Therapists often forget to take care of themselves, some simple self-massage techniques will help to reduce stress on the body (see pages 113–115).

THE HEARING-IMPAIRED CLIENT

If you are treating a hearing-impaired client your massage style will not change but your body language and pre-post care will. You need to be able engage their attention, which can be done by eye contact or by tapping them lightly on the shoulder. Anything that your client does not understand may need to be rephrased rather than repeated and if your client lip reads, enunciated normally. Be expressive with your face and body to communicate. If your client is wearing a hearing aid, avoid moving your hands close to it as this may produce feedback. Before you start, agree a signal for your client to indicate that the pressure of the massage is tolerable. Above all, do not forget that it is only the client's hearing that is impaired, not their intelligence.

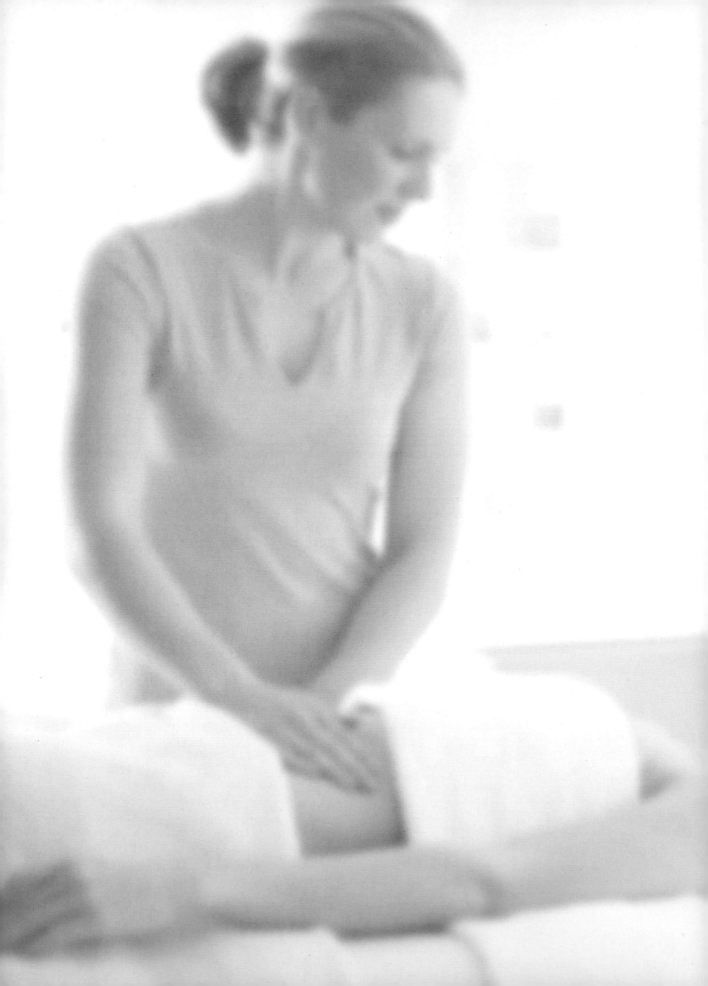

The body and the effects of massage

Study of human anatomy (structure) and physiology (function) is intrinsic to a massage therapist's training. If you are to become a professional and skilful therapist, you must have a comprehensive knowledge of the subject and be able to navigate your way around the body confidently. Studies are commonly broken down into ten systems: skeletal (bones and joints), muscular, digestive, circulatory (cardiovascular and lymphatic), nervous, reproductive, respiratory, endocrine, urinary and integumentary (hair, skin and nails). This chapter is meant as a simple guide, highlighting the systems that your training will cover in depth.

Terminology

Although most people have some basic knowledge from personal experience about how the body works and how it is constructed, for the therapist this knowledge needs to be defined within a medically based common language.

Because of its Latin and Greek terminology, the language of medicine is often the most daunting aspect of an entry-level massage course, but once you understand and begin to visualize what happens beneath your hands as massage is applied, the language will become easier as the subject becomes more fascinating.

Before the individual systems are addressed, the terms used to locate positions within the body need to be learned.

Anatomical terms

As the human is a three-dimensional structure, it can be divided into three parts or planes, known as the planes of reference:

- **Sagittal or medial plane** – runs vertically through the body from top to bottom dividing the whole body into left and right parts.
- **Frontal or coronal plane** – runs vertically from left to right dividing body into front and back parts.
- **Transverse or horizontal plane** – runs through the middle of the body, dividing it into top and bottom parts.

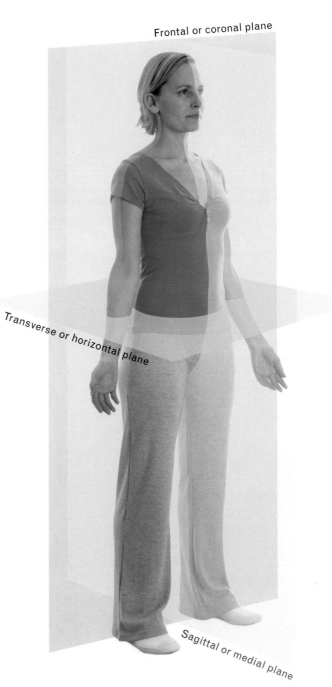

Frontal or coronal plane

Transverse or horizontal plane

Sagittal or medial plane

Other terms that you will use regularly are:

- **Anatomical position** – The body in a standing position, feet parallel and about hip distance, arms at side, palms of hands forward and pointing downwards.
- **Anterior** – To the front of another structure (e.g. the nose is anterior to the cheek).
- **Posterior** – To the back (e.g. the cheek is posterior to the nose).
- **Superior** – Above (towards the head) (e.g. the lips are superior to the chin).
- **Inferior** – Below (e.g. the chin is inferior to the lips).
- **Medial** – Towards the midline of the body (e.g. the navel is medial).
- **Lateral** – Towards the side (e.g. the ribs are lateral to the vertebral column).
- **Proximal** – Nearest to the point of reference (e.g. the proximal end of a bone is the end furthest from its origin).
- **Distal** – Furthest from the point of reference.
- **Supine** – Facing upwards (lying on the back with face, palms, feet up).
- **Prone** – Facing downwards (lying on the front with face, palms, feet down).

For example, elevating and depressing the mandible (jaw bone) opens and closes the mouth; retracting and protracting the mandible juts the lower jaw in and out.

Two other less commonly used terms are *lateral flexion/deviation*, which is a side-to-side movement, and *opposition*, in which the tip of a thumb contacts the tip of any other digit on the same hand.

Finally other relevant structures you will need to have knowledge of when studying the anatomy are:

- **Muscle** – Attached to two articulating bones, contraction of muscles leads to movement. Muscles pass across a joint and attach to the bones that form the joint. The place where the muscle attaches to a relatively stationary point on a bone is called the *origin*, the end of the muscle that moves with the bone is known as the *insertion*.
- **Tendon** – A band of connective tissue that attaches muscle to bone.
- **Ligament** – A band of connective tissue that holds together two bones at a joint, reinforcing the joint capsule and limiting movement.
- **Bursa** – A fluid-filled sac that cushions the movement of bone over other tissues or tendons.

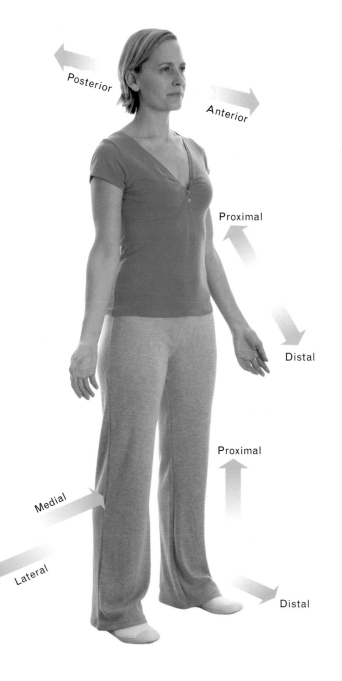

Movement terminology

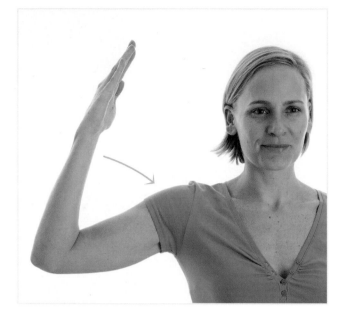

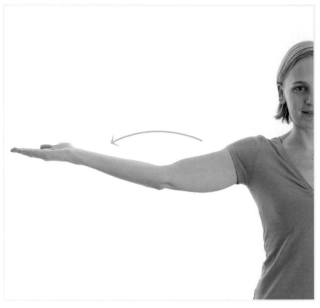

Flexion – Any forward (anterior) movement away from the anatomical position. Bending of a joint, decreasing the angle of the bones (e.g. bending the arm at the elbow or curling the fingers). The exception is flexion of the knee or toes, which is a backward movement.

Extension – The reverse of flexion, returning to the anatomical position. Increasing the angle of the joints (e.g. straightening the arm at the elbow or uncurling the fingers). Hyperextension is when the angle extends beyond the anatomical position.

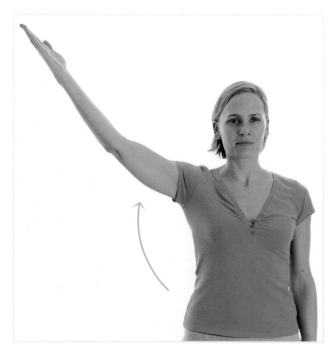

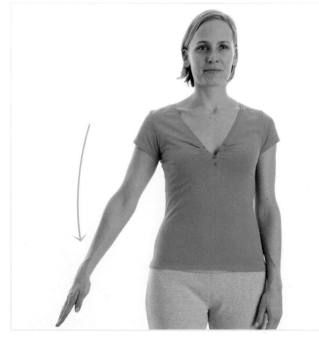

Abduction – A lateral movement away from the midline of the body (e.g. lifting the arms sideways).

Adduction – Reverse of abduction, movement towards the midline of the body (e.g. lowering the arms sideways).

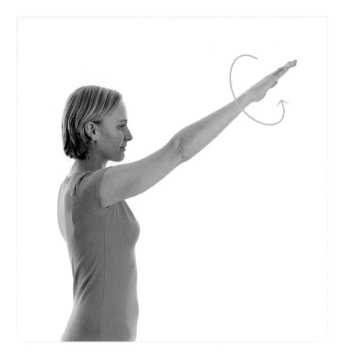

Circumduction – A circular motion of a body part combining flexion, extension, abduction and adduction (e.g. drawing a circle with a straight arm).

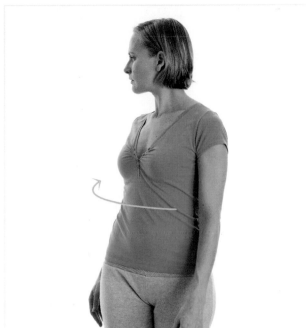

Rotation – A bone moves around its own axis in a circular movement (e.g. turning the head or moving the trunk from side to side).

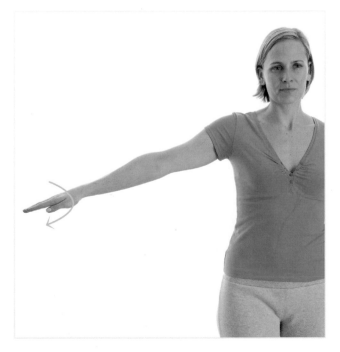

Pronation – Medial rotation of the forearm that brings the palm of the hand from upward facing to downward facing position.

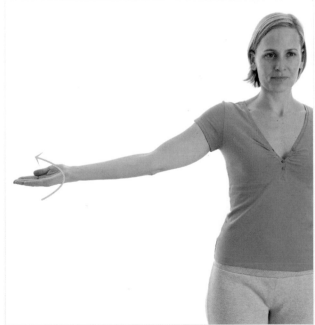

Supination – Reverse of pronation, bringing the palm of the hand from a downward to an upward facing position.

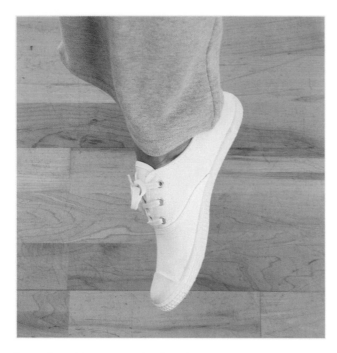

Inversion – Turning the sole of the foot inward.

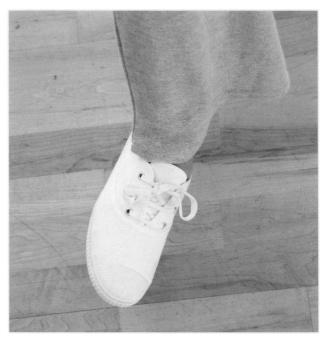

Eversion – Reverse of inversion, turning sole of the foot outwards.

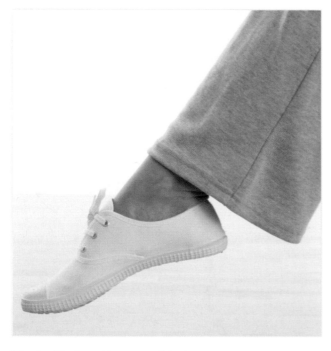

Plantar flexion – Extension of the foot past the anatomical position (e.g. walking on tiptoe).

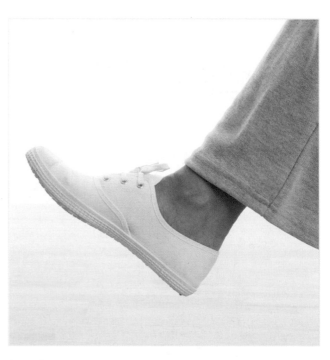

Dorsiflexion – Flexing the ankle dorsally (e.g. walking on the heels).

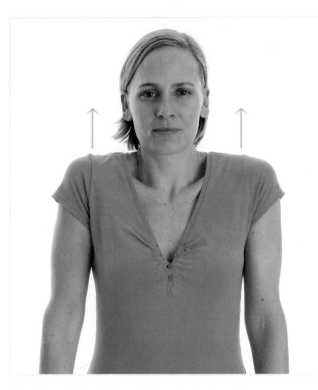

Elevation – The raising or lifting of a body part in a superior direction.

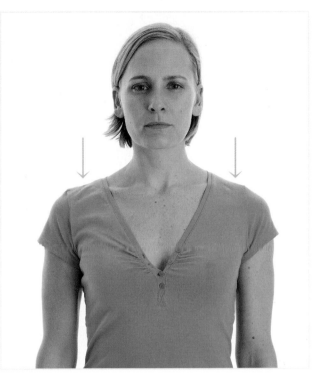

Depression – Reverse of elevation, lowering a body part inferiorly.

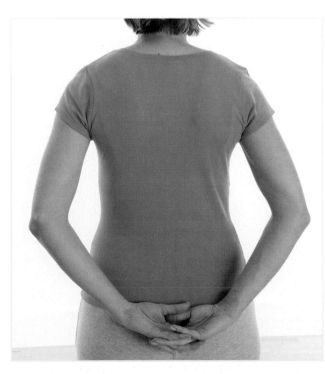

Protraction – Moving the bone forward or anteriorly.

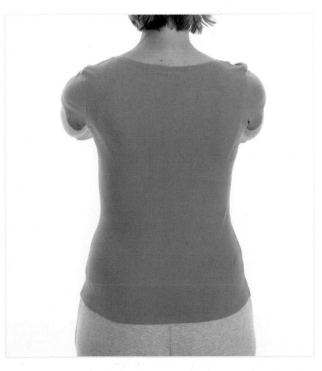

Retraction – Reverse of protraction, moving backwards or posteriorly.

Cells and tissues

The body is made up of cells of many different types, each with a specific purpose and function, such as blood cells or nerve cells. When grouped together according to structure or function they form tissue, such as muscle or bone.

Cell types

The simplest form of self-sustaining life, cells are the building blocks of the body. They divide to form genetically identical or 'daughter' cells, in the process known as mitosis. There are estimated to be around 50 trillion cells in an adult and 26 billion in a newborn baby.

The size and shape of each cell is related to the specific functions it perform. In general, a cell consists of:

- **Cytoplasm** – a jelly-like mass that contains a great variety of substances needed by the cell.
- **Cell membrane** – a thin membrane surrounding the cell, protecting it and regulating the passage of materials in and out. The cell is nourished through the cell membrane.
- **Nucleus** – the control centre that contains the 46 chromosomes that hold the genetic information or DNA of the cell.
- **Organelles** – small organs scattered throughout the cytoplasm that perform specific functions, they store and transport food and manufacture substances in the cell.

In some areas of the body, such as the lining of the respiratory tract, the cells also have tiny hair-like processes on their surfaces called cilia. These help move materials which are outside the cell.

There are over 200 distinct types of cell in the human body, including cells designed for secretion or storage, cells that cause movement, cells involved in the immune system, cells that transmit messages and cells that fill in the gaps. Each cell type has a size and shape appropriate to its function.

Epithelial cells resemble building blocks. They join to form tissues that cover the body surfaces and line body cavities. They can be flat, cuboid or column-shaped, depending on where they are situated. Sometimes they have a secretory function.

Nerve cells, often referred to as neurons, have long extensions and specialize in transmitting messages from one part of the body to another.

Lymphocytes, or white blood cells, move through the tissues of the body, destroying invading bacteria and playing a vitally important role in the workings of the immune system.

Muscle cells are specialized to aid contraction and can move externally. In the body there are three types of muscle tissue: skeletal muscles attached to bones, cardiac muscle in the heart (control is involuntary) and smooth muscle that occurs in the digestive tract (control is involuntary).

The cell membrane

The membrane surrounding a cell has an important function in regulating the passage of substances such as oxygen, water and nutrients in and out of the cell. Transport across the cell membrane is either active or passive. In active transport the molecules are moved against the concentration gradient using energy in the form of ATP. In passive transport substances move down a gradient, either by diffusion from an area of high concentration to low concentration or, in the case of water, by osmosis.

It is important for the body to maintain its homeostasis, or the 'state of being the same', by adapting to different environments. The cell membrane has an important role in this, helping the cells to regulate body temperature, blood sugar levels, metabolism, water and mineral levels.

Body tissues

A group of cells with a specific function is called a tissue and there are four main types: epithelial, connective, muscle and nervous. The study of tissues is known as histology.

- **Epithelial tissue** is a lining or covering that protects surfaces. It can be made up of a single row of cells or several layers. Examples are the linings of the digestive tract, the respiratory tract and the kidney tubules. The shapes of the cells in the epithelial tissue can be flat, cube-like or tall and rectangular and during sleep they

Cell The basic unit of all living organisms can reproduce itself exactly. Each cell is bounded by a cell membrane of lipids and proteins that controls the passage of substances in and out of the cell.

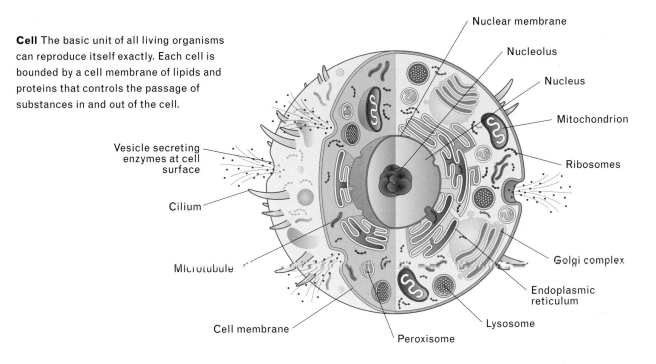

Nuclear membrane

Nucleolus

Nucleus

Mitochondrion

Ribosomes

Golgi complex

Endoplasmic reticulum

Lysosome

Peroxisome

Cell membrane

Microtubule

Cilium

Vesicle secreting enzymes at cell surface

reproduce more rapidly, encouraging growth and tissue repair.

- **Connective tissue** joins together other tissues to support the body's structure. Examples are fat or adipose tissue, cartilage, bone and blood. Connective tissue is separated by a dense mesh of collagen, elastic and support or reticular fibres. The structure of this mesh determines whether the connective tissue is soft, firm or rigid.

For the massage therapist a knowledge of a type of connective tissue known as *fascia* is important. Tension of the superficial fascia immediately below the skin and the deep fascia that covers muscles is addressed through massage. As the fascia warms up, it loosens and becomes more flexible, allowing the muscles it protects to be manipulated and also relax, no longer restricted by a tight casing.

- **Muscle tissue** is able to produce movement. It can shorten or contract, has elasticity and can respond to nerve impulses. Examples are the smooth muscle of the digestive tract, which helps to push food along, the cardiac muscle of the heart, contracting rhythmically approximately 100,000 a day, and the skeletal muscles, attached to bone, of which there are over 600 throughout the body. A good example of the range of movements possible is the face, the muscles of which allow us to produce an enormous variety of facial expressions.

- **Nervous tissue** is found in the brain, spinal cord and nerves. It is made up of cells called neurons that can receive and transmit messages through nerve impulses. Nervous tissue can control muscles and glands and coordinates the body processes by stimulating a response to changes both internally and externally.

Body membranes

Body membranes are thin sheets of tissue that cover or line body surfaces to provide protection and support. They also divide the body into regions and facilitate movement. Some also produce their own secretions.

Membranes can be classified as epithelial or connective tissue. There are three types of epithelial membranes:

- **Cutaneous** – more commonly known as the skin.
- **Mucous** – lines cavities open to the environment and secretes mucus to lubricate the surface.
- **Serous** – found within the body, such as the thoracic and abdominal cavities.
  Connective tissue membranes are:
- **Synovial** – lines joint cavities such as those of the shoulder, knee and hip and secrete synovial fluid to lubricate and assist free movement of the joints.
- **Meninges** – the connective tissue membrane that covers the brain and spinal cord and although does not produce fluid, when inflamed or infected is a life-threatening condition.

Bones

For the therapist, bones are the natural pathways used to locate muscle and soft tissue attached at points called origins and insertions. A special form of connective tissue, bone consists of compact tissue, spongy cancellous tissue, collagenous fibres and mineral salts.

The human skeleton contains 206 major bones divided into two distinct types: *axial* bones are associated with the central axis and *appendicular* bones are associated with the extremities. The skeleton has five main functions:

- **Support** – It serves as a supporting framework for the body, in effect its internal scaffolding.
- **Protection** – It shields the major organs (e.g. the ribcage protects the heart and lungs).
- **Movement** – The bones and their joints act as levers, powered by muscle to create movement.
- **Storage** – Vital minerals such as calcium and phosphorus and fats are stored in cavities of the bone and act as reservoirs to be called upon when required.
- **Production** – Red and white blood cells are produced in the red bone marrow.

There are five types of bone based on their shape:

- **Long** – The length is greater than the width (e.g. humerus).
- **Short** – The length, width and depth are similar (e.g. tarsals).
- **Flat** – Broad and flat, for attachment and protective purposes (e.g. shoulder blade).
- **Irregular** – All bones that do not fit other classifications (e.g. vertebrae).
- **Sesamoid** – Small, round bones developed in tendons (e.g. patella).

BONES OF THE AXIAL SKELETON

SKULL OR CRANIUM
29 bones consisting of: 8 Cranial (frontal, nasal, orbit, maxilla, mandible, zygomatic, parietal, occipital) (F), 14 Facial (I), 6 Ear ossicles (I), 1 Hyoid (Se)

VERTEBRAL COLUMN
26 bones consisting of: 24 Vertebrae (I), 1 sacrum (I), 1 Coccyx (I)

THORACIC CAGE
25 bones consisting of: 24 Ribs (F), 1 Sternum (F)

L = long; S = short; F = flat; I = irregular; Se = sesamoid

BONES OF THE APPENDICULAR SKELETON

PECTORAL OR SHOULDER GIRDLE
4 bones consisting of: 2 Clavicles (L), 2 Scapula (F)

UPPER LIMBS
60 bones consisting of: 2 Humerus (L), 2 Radius (L), 2 Ulna (L), 16 Carpals (S), 10 Metacarpals (L), 28 Phalanges (L)

PELVIC GIRDLE
2 bones consisting of: 2 Coxa or hip (ischium, ilium, pubis fused together) (F)

LOWER LIMBS
60 bones consisting of: 2 Femur (L), 2 Patella (Se), 2 Tibia (L), 2 Fibula (L), 14 Tarsals (S), 10 Metatarsals (L), 28 Phalanges (L)

L = long; S = short; F = flat; I = irregular; Se = sesamoid

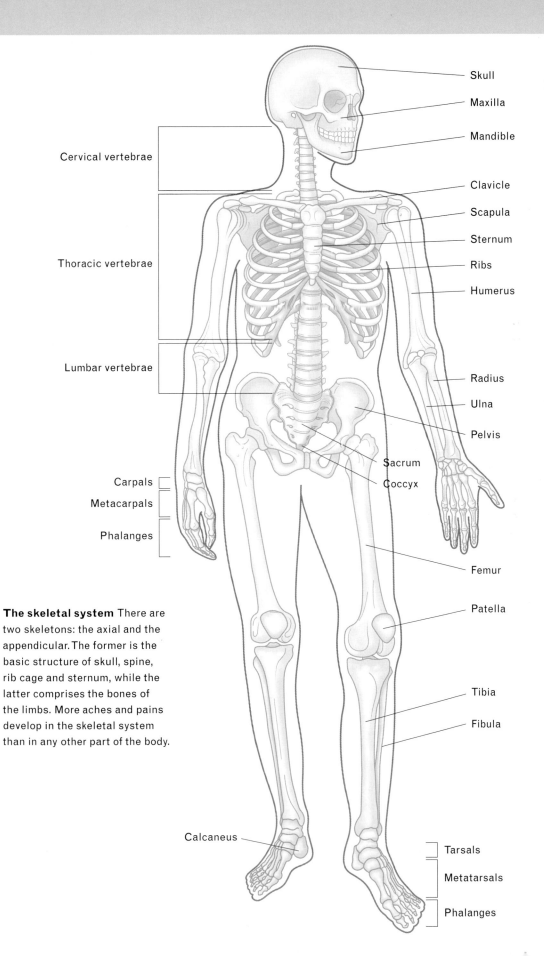

Skull

Maxilla

Mandible

Clavicle

Scapula

Sternum

Ribs

Humerus

Radius

Ulna

Pelvis

Cervical vertebrae

Thoracic vertebrae

Lumbar vertebrae

Sacrum

Coccyx

Carpals

Metacarpals

Phalanges

Femur

Patella

Tibia

Fibula

The skeletal system There are two skeletons: the axial and the appendicular. The former is the basic structure of skull, spine, rib cage and sternum, while the latter comprises the bones of the limbs. More aches and pains develop in the skeletal system than in any other part of the body.

Calcaneus

Tarsals

Metatarsals

Phalanges

Joints

Whereas bones provide a solid framework to which muscles are attached, joints or articulations, as they are sometimes called, enable movement. Joints are formed where two or more bones meet and come in a variety of forms, determined by their style and range of movement.

Problems with joints occur when they are used in a way they were not designed for. For example the wrist joint is not loadbearing and if too much weight is placed on a flexed wrist it gets injured. A common injury is a broken wrist as a result of a fall. The natural reflex as you fall is to put out a hand for stabilization, which means the wrist joint takes the full impact.

There is a relationship between the stability of a joint and its articulation – the more secure and solid the joint, the less mobile it is. The shoulder joint has the most flexibility. To allow this it is seated in a shallow socket, resulting in a higher incidence of injury than, say, the hip joint which sits in a deeper socket and has a more limited type and range of movement.

Types of joints

Joints fall into three classifications depending on their range of motion:

- **Synarthrosis or fibrous** – These are immobile joints, held together by fibrous tissue or cartilage. They are found in the skull (sutures) and the connection of a tooth to its socket.
- **Amphiarthroses or cartilaginous** – These are slightly movable joints and fall into two categories: in *primary* or *syndesmosis* joints the two bones are held together by cartilage (e.g. the tibia and fibula joint just below the knee) whereas in *secondary* or *symphysis* joints the bone ends are covered by cartilage and in between the ends is a disc of fibrocartilage (e.g. the anterior ends of the pubic bones).
- **Diarthroses or synovial** – These are freely movable joints. There are six types. Most of the body's joints are synovial (e.g. toes, knees, hips, shoulders, elbows and wrists).

Synovial joints differ from other types of joint in that the space between the bones of the joint, known as the joint cavity, is filled with a lubricant called synovial fluid. This allows the bones to move smoothly past each other,

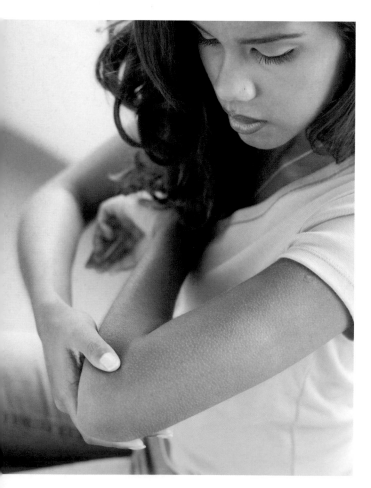

The elbow This is a hinge joint of the bones of the upper and lower arm, allowing the arm to flex and extend.

SYNOVIAL JOINTS

BALL AND SOCKET

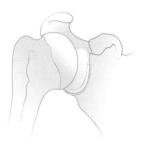

DESCRIPTION
A round ball fits into a concave, cup-shaped socket, allowing it to move around many axes

EXAMPLES
Hip and shoulder joints

TYPE OF MOVEMENT
Flexion, extension, abduction, adduction, rotation, circumduction

GLIDING

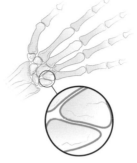

DESCRIPTION
The articular surfaces glide over each other, allowing movement around many axes

EXAMPLES
Carpal and tarsal joints

TYPE OF MOVEMENT
Flat gliding

SADDLE

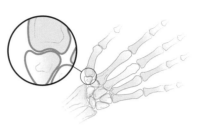

DESCRIPTION
Each joint surface is both concave and convex and fits into its opposite of the other bone surface (i.e. saddle-shaped), allowing movement around two axes

EXAMPLES
Carpometacarpal joint of the thumb

TYPE OF MOVEMENT
Flexion, extension, abduction, adduction, rotation, circumduction

ELLIPSOID OR CONDYLOID

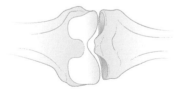

DESCRIPTION
Two convex oval surfaces fit into two concave oval surfaces, allowing movements around two axes rather like a restricted ball and socket joint

EXAMPLES
Wrist

TYPE OF MOVEMENT
Flexion, extension, abduction, adduction

HINGE

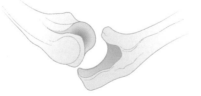

DESCRIPTION
The convex surface of one bone fits into the concave surface of another, allowing movement in one axis in a hinge action

EXAMPLES
Elbow and ankle

TYPE OF MOVEMENT
Flexion and extension

PIVOT

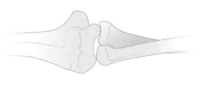

DESCRIPTION
A small projection of one bone pivots in a ring-shaped socket of another bone allowing movement in one axis

EXAMPLES
Joint between the first (atlas) and second vertebrae (axis)

TYPE OF MOVEMENT
Pivoting

rather like oil in an engine. A layer of hyaline cartilage covers each bone at the joint, acting as a shock absorber to absorb impact. This whole construction is then held together by a fibrous capsule of connective tissue lined with a synovial membrane.

The names of the synovial joints are descriptive of their shape or movement and are therefore easy to remember.

The important synovial joints in the appendicular skeleton are shown in the box below.

Effects of massage on bones and joints

Although massage does not have an effect on the bones or joints themselves, it does affect problems surrounding them relating to the fascia, muscles, tendons, bursae and ligaments. Tension is transmitted to the bone through the connective tissue so it is the effect of massage on the

tissue that indirectly affects the bones and joints. The range of motion of joints and bones can be improved with specific techniques that prevent adhesions, together with the use of passive stretching and mobilization movements.

Massage for common conditions of the bones and joints

When you are practising as a massage therapist you will come across re-occurring problems relating to bones and joints, which clients wish you to address. Some of these conditions are discussed here. It is important to remember that although massage cannot correct bone deformities it can help alleviate the related problems.

Ankylosing spondylitis

This is a condition resulting from progressive loss of range of movement due to the calcification and ossification of the spine.

Massage: Place the client in a comfortable position. Do not force the problem joint into any movement. Apply techniques that will maintain joint mobility.

Kyphosis, scoliosis and lordosis

These are deformities of the spine. In kyphosis the back is rounded, in scoliosis the deformity is lateral and in lordosis the spine curves forward abnormally, forming a pronounced concavity of the lower back.

Massage: If using movements, be careful not to overstretch the spine. The massage should focus on the supporting muscles of the pectoralis, rhomboids and serratus anterior.

Osteoarthritis and rheumatoid arthritis

Both of these are painful conditions. Osteoarthritis is the result of wear and tear on the articular cartilage, which produces chronic inflammation and is common in the weight-bearing joints of the elderly. Rheumatoid arthritis affects all ages and is believed to be an autoimmune disease that destroys synovial membranes, reducing range of movement. Commonly affecting the joints of the hands and feet, the painful symptoms come and go depending on the degree of inflammation.

Massage: Apply light techniques on the surrounding tissues to warm and reduce tension. With rheumatoid arthritis, massage is contraindicated when symptoms have flared up; for osteoarthritis, mobilizations and deep stretching are also contraindicated.

Osteoporosis

This disorder is common in postmenopausal women because the lower levels of oestrogen reduce the rate of

THE IMPORTANT SYNOVIAL JOINTS FOUND IN THE APPENDICULAR SKELETON

	Type of joint
The shoulder girdle	
Acromioclavicular	Gliding
Sternoclavicular	Ball and socket
The upper limb	
Shoulder	Ball and socket
Elbow	Hinge
Radio-ulnar, proximal and distal	Pivot
Wrist	Ellipsoid
Intercarpal	Gliding
Carpometacarpal	Gliding
Metacarpophalangeal	Ellipsoid or condyloid
Interphalangeal	Hinge
The lower limb	
Hip	Ball and socket
Knee	Ellipsoid or condyloid
Tibiofubular, proximal and distal	Pivot
Ankle	Hinge
Tarsal and metatarsals	Gliding
Metatarsophalangeal	Ellipsoid or condyloid
Interphalangeal	Hinge

calcium replenishment in the bone. This weakens the skeleton and increases the risk of fracture, particularly in the vertebral column and hip.

Massage: Due to the fragility of the bones, only apply light pressure. Always check with the client during treatment and avoid mobilization of any kind.

Bursitis

Inflammation of the bursa, a fluid-filled sac that cushions the movement of bone over other tissues, is a painful condition. The elbows and knees are most commonly affected. The large bursa under the deltoid of the shoulder is also prone to bursitis, which will cause pain on abducting the arm.

Massage: While the condition is acute massage is contraindicated, but application of cool packs or ice applied to the area can bring some relief. When it becomes suitable to massage, use friction, mobilization and stretching to help maintain joint mobility. As with whiplash conditions, end the massage session by cooling the treated area.

Fractures

There are three main types of bone fracture: simple, compound and stress. Simple fractures are closed and do not break the skin; they could even be a partial break or crack such as a greenstick fracture, where the bone is partly bent and only splinters on the convex side. In a compound fracture the bone pierces the skin or communicates with an open wound. Stress fractures are the result of repetitive mechanical stress, usually found in the leg as a result of running on a hard surface.

Massage: Once the client has clinical confirmation that the fracture has healed, massage can be applied to help increase tone in the surrounding muscle and to aid increase in mobility. Work within the client's comfort zone. If the client is having problems with circulation, pain and water retention while the fracture is still healing, massage is only suitable in the surrounding areas, working proximal and then distal to the affected area. This will help the healing process as increased circulation leads to increased deposits of callus to the bone.

Frozen shoulder

Also known as adhesive capsulitis, this condition is very painful and severely reduces range of movement due to the tightening of the joint capsule.

Neck pain A modern day complaint affecting the muscles of the neck and reducing range of movement is the repetitive strain caused by constant use of a mobile phone.

Massage: Stretching and mobilization techniques applied in the early stages of the condition can help, working within the tolerance of the client. If the condition has been left too long without attention, referral to an osteopath is recommended.

Whiplash

This condition occurs when the head and neck are thrown forcefully back and forth as in a car collision. It is called whiplash because the lower three vertebrae of the cervical spine act like the handle of a whip, which then lashes the upper four vertebrae, causing strain or a sprain of the cervical spine and spinal cord.

Massage: Until the client has medical clearance, massage is contraindicated. Once massage is approved, establish whether the whiplash was lateral or anterior/posterior. For lateral whiplash work on the sternocleidomastoid and scalenes; for anterior/posterior whiplash focus also on the levator scapula, upper trapezius and splenius muscles. End the session by applying a cold pack or cool gel to the area.

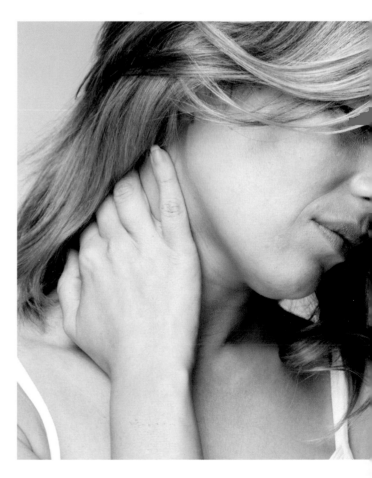

Muscles

The muscular system is the workhorse of the body; all functions of the body that involve movement, from standing to breathing to pumping blood require muscle power. This system is the primary focus for a massage therapist and the comprehensive knowledge required is often at a higher level than that needed by other health practitioners.

It is not enough to rely on a knowledge of what each muscle consists of and how it works. The massage therapist must learn and be familiar with the individual muscle attachments (origin and insertion) for each part of the body in order that dysfunctional conditions can be addressed. In sports massage the maintenance of the muscular system plays an important role in injury prevention and management, as well as in maximizing efficiency and skills.

Muscles are classified as involuntary or voluntary. Involuntary muscles cannot be controlled at will, they move automatically in response to messages from the brain. Heart muscle, for example, is an involuntary muscle. Voluntary muscles are under conscious control and can be made to contract whenever we want to move. They are arranged in layers, symmetrically on each side of the body and tend to work in groups.

Origins, insertions and actions

As a therapist you will need to know all the main muscle groups and the origins, insertions and actions of each. Because muscles work from the insertion (where the muscle is attached to the moving bone) to the origin (the fixed point), the general rule is to massage in the same direction to achieve maximum benefit. As you gain experience, you will also come across pain located around the origin of a muscle that may be caused by a problem around its insertion point.

Muscle is attached by tendons to a bone at each end:

- The *origin* is at the fixed end of the muscle. It hardly moves and is located closest to the midline (proximal).
- The *insertion* is the moving end of the muscle and is usually the furthest away from the midline (distal).
- The *action* is the change that occurs to a joint when the muscle contracts. This action or movement and its direction can be identified by the origin and insertion of the muscle.

Agonists and antagonists, synergists and fixators

Muscles function in a variety of ways depending on the role played in a specific action. As they often work in

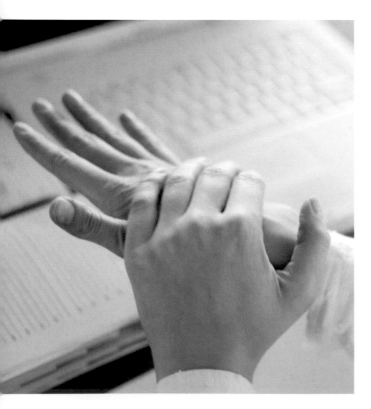

Wrist and hand There are seven main muscle groups whose actions facilitate the movement of the wrist and hand, and maintain a range of motion.

pairs and lie on opposite sides of a joint, they will work in an opposing manner. For example, in order to flex the muscles of the forearm, the biceps contract and so are the prime mover or *agonist*, whereas the triceps in the back of the forearm extend in order to allow this action and so act as the *antagonists*. Muscles that help the agonist are called *synergists* and those that help stabilize the joint are called *fixators*.

Naming the muscles

It may seem a daunting task to learn the names of the muscles but once you grasp the logic to the labelling you will find it easier than you think. Any muscle that has *brevis* in its name is a small muscle (as in brief); *serratus* means saw-toothed (as in serrated); *maximus* is the biggest and *minimus* the smallest. Bring some fun into studying by introducing bodybuilding magazines – a great learning aid with photographs of well-defined muscles to locate and name.

The following tables show the major muscles, their origins, insertions and functions. These are often taught in sections of the body, but here we have listed them in areas of movement.

MUSCLES OF THE SHOULDER MOVEMENT

	ORIGIN	INSERTION	ACTION
Coracobrachialis	Scapula – coracoid process	Humerus – middle	Flexes arm
Deltoid	Clavicle	Humerus – deltoid tuberosity	Flexes and extends arm
	Scapula – spine and acromion process		Abducts arm
			Medial and lateral rotation of arm
Latissimus dorsi	Scapula – inferior angle	Humerus – bicipital groove	Extends arm
	Lumbar and thoracic (T7–T12) vertebrae		Adducts arm
	Sacrum and iliac crest		Medially rotates arm
Pectoralis major	Clavicle	Humerus – lateral lip of bicipital groove	Flexes and adducts arm
	Sternum		Medial rotates arm
Teres major	Scapula – inferior angle	Humerus – medial lip of bicipital groove	Extends, adducts and medially rotates arm
Known as the rotator cuff:			
Infraspinatus	Scapula	Humerus and capsule of shoulder joint	Supports, stabilizes, strengthens shoulder joint
Subscapularis	Scapula	Humerus and front of shoulder capsule	Supports, stabilizes, strengthens shoulder joint
Supraspinatus	Scapula	Humerus and capsule of shoulder joint	Supports, stabilizes, strengthens shoulder joint
Teres minor	Scapula	Humerus and capsule of shoulder joint	Supports, stabilizes, strengthens shoulder joint

MUSCLES OF ELBOW AND FOREARM MOVEMENT

	ORIGIN	INSERTION	ACTION
Biceps brachii	Scapula – supraglenoid tubercle and coracoid	Radius – radial tuberosity	Flexes and supinates forearm, supinates hand
Brachialis	Humerus – anterior – crosses elbow	Ulna – proximal	Flexes forearm
Brachioradialis	Humerus – condyloid ridge	Radius – distal	Flexes forearm
Pronator teres	Humerus – above medial epicondyle	Radius	Pronates and flexes forearm and hand
Pronator quadratus	Ulna – shaft	Radius	Pronates weakly the forearm and hand
Supinator	Humerus – lateral epicondyle	Radius	Supinates forearm and hand
Triceps brachii	Humerus – medial and lateral head. Scapula – long head	Ulna	Extends forearm
Anconeus	Humerus – lateral epicondyle	Ulna – olecranon process	Extends elbow
Flexor carpi radialis	Humerus – medial epicondyle	2nd and 3rd metacarpal bones	Flexes and abducts wrist

MUSCLES OF THE HEAD AND NECK MOVEMENT

	ORIGIN	INSERTION	ACTION
Buccinator	Maxillae and Mandible	Cheeks	Compresses cheek
Frontalis	Connective tissue covering scalp	Skin of eyebrow and bridge of nose	Wrinkes forehead, raises eyebrows
Masseter	Zygomatic arch	Mandible – lateral surface	Elevates mandible
Occipitalis	Superior nuchal	Galea aponeurosis	Tenses and draws back scalp
Orbicularis oculi and oris	Orbit – medial margin	Skin around eyelid	Closes eye
Pterygoid medial and lateral	Roof of mouth – lateral aspect	Mandible – medial surface	Moves mandible side to side, elevates and protracts
Scalenes anterior, medius and posterior	Cervical vertebrae – transverse process	1st and 2nd rib – superior surface	Flexes neck, elevates ribs
Sternocleidomastoid	Sternum, clavicle	Mastoid process, occipital bone	Flexes and rotates neck
Temporalis	Along the temple	Mandible – coronoid process	Elevates mandible
Zygomaticus major and minor	Zygomatic bone	Angle of mouth	Moves corner of mouth back and upwards

Other muscles in the head and neck are:
Longus capitis, Longus colli, Oblique capitis superior and inferior, Platysma, Rectus capitis posterior major and minor, Splenius capitis and cervicis

MUSCLES OF WRIST AND HAND MOVEMENT

	ORIGIN	INSERTION	ACTION
Extensor carpi radialis longus and brevis	Humerus – lateral epicondyle	Base of 2nd and 3rd metacarpals	Extends and abducts palm of hand
Extensor carpi ulnaris	Humerus – lateral epicondyle	Base of 5th metacarpal	Extends and abducts palm of hand
Extensor digitorum	Humerus – lateral epicondyle	Phalanges – dorsal surface	Extends fingers
Flexor carpi radialis	Humerus – medial epicondyle	Base of 3rd and 4th metacarpals	Extends and abducts palm of hand
Flexor carpi ulnaris	Humerus – medial epicondyle and ulna	Base of 3rd and 4th metacarpals	Flexes and adducts palm of hand
Flexor digitorum superficialis and profundus	Humerus – medial epicondyle	2nd phalanx of fingers and base of distal	Flexes fingers and palm of hand
Palmaris longus	Humerus – medial epicondyle	Variable/Palmar Aponeurosis	Flexes wrist

Other muscles used in wrist and hand functions are:
Abductor longus and brevis, Digiti minimi extensor, flexor, abductor and opponens, Extensor indicis, Extensor and flexor pollicis longus and brevis, Opponens pollicis

MUSCLES OF TRUNK AND VERTEBRAL COLUMN MOVEMENT

	ORIGIN	INSERTION	ACTION
Erector spinae	Iliac crest, sacrum	Occipital bone	Extension and lateral bening of vertebral column
Obliques external and internal	Iliac crest, lower 8 costal cartilages (ribs)	Linea alba and iliac crest	Depresses ribs, lateraly flexes and rotates spine
Quadratus lumborum	Iliac crest	12th rib and transerve process of lumbar vertebrae	Depresses ribs, flexes spine
Rectus abdominis	Symphysis pubis	Lower ribs, xiphoid process	Depresses ribs, flexes spine
Transverse abdominis	Iliac crest, lower 6 costal artilages (ribs)	Linea alba and pubus iliac crest	Compresses abdomen
Iliocostalis lumborum	Iliac crest	Lower 7 ribs – inferior	Extends spine, lowers ribs
Longissimus	Lower thoracic vertebrae – transverse process	Ribs – inferior, upper transverse process	Extends and bends spine
Multifidus	Transverse process of vertebrae and sacrum	Spinous process of vertebrae, 5 above origin	Extends and rotates vertebrae

Other muscles in the trunk and vertebral column are:
Paraspinals, Rotatores, Spinalis, semi and transverso

MUSCLES OF PULMONARY RESPIRATION

	ORIGIN	INSERTION	ACTION
Diaphragm	Sternum – xiphoid process, lower ribs, lumbar vertebrae	Central tendon	Inceases volume of thoracic capacity
Intercostal internal and external	Superior and inferior borders of ribs	Superior surface of each rib below	Raises and depresses ribs, expands and contracts thorax
Serratus posterior superior and inferior	Upper nine ribs	Scapula – anterior of vertebral border	Draws shoulder forward with abduction of scapula

MUSCLES OF HIP AND KNEE MOVEMENT

	ORIGIN	INSERTION	ACTION
Adductors longus, magnus and brevis – adductors	Pubis	Femur shaft – posterior	Adducts and laterally rotates thigh
Biceps femoris	Ischium tuberosity	Tibia – lateral condyle and fibula head	Extends thigh and flexes leg at knee
Gluteus maximus – rotators	Ilium and sacrum	Femur – proximal iliotibial tract	Extends and rotates hip joint, extends trunk
Gluteus medius and minimus – abductors and rotators	Ilium	Femur – greater trochanter	Abducts and medially rotates thigh
Gracilis – adductors	Pubis	Tibia – medial condyle	Adducts thigh, flexes leg
Iliopsoas-psoas major and iliacus	Iliac fossa, T12 and lumbar vertebrae	Femur – lesser trochanter	Flexes hip and verterbral column
Pectineus – adductors	Pubis	Femur – lesser trochanter	Adducts, flexes and medially rotates thigh
Piriformis	Front of sacrum	Femur – greater trochanter	Rotates laterally the hip
Rectus femoris – quadriceps	Superior acetabulum rim	Tibial tuberosity	Extends leg, flexes thigh
Sartorius	Ilium – anterior superior spine	Tibia – medial condyle	Flexes, abducts, laterally rotates thigh. Flexes leg at knee
Semimembranosus	Ischium tuberosity	Tibia – medial condyle	Extends thigh, medially rotates leg, flexes leg at knee
Semitendinosus	Ischium tuberosity	Tibia – medial condyle	Extends thigh, medially rotates leg, flexes leg at knee
Tensor fascia lata	Ilium crest	Iliotibial tract on upper thigh	Flexes and medially rotates thigh
Vastus intermedius, medialis and lateralis – quadriceps	Femur shaft, linea alba, greater trochanter	Tibial tuberosity	Extends leg

Other muscles used in hip and knee functions are:
Gemellus superior and inferior, Obturator externus and internus, Pes anserinus, Popliteus

MUSCLES OF ANKLE AND FOOT MOVEMENT

	ORIGIN	INSERTION	ACTION
Extensor digitorum longus and brevis	Tibia and fibula – proximal	2, 3, 4 and 5 phalanges	Flexes toes, assists plantar flexion and inverts foot
Flexor digitorum longus	Tibia – posterior surface	2, 3, 4 and 5 phalanges	Flexes toes, assists plantar flexion and inverts foot
Gastrocnemius	Femur – lateral and medial condyles	Calcaneus – by Achilles tendon	Flexes leg at knee, assists plantar flexion of foot
Peroneus longus and brevis	Tibia – lateral condyle, fibula – head	Base of 1st metatarsal	Plantar flexion and eversion of foot
Peroneus tertius	Fibula – distal	5th metatarsal	Dorsiflexion and eversion of foot
Plantaris soleus	Tibia and fibula – proximal	Calcaneus – by Achilles tendon	Plantar flexion of foot
Tibialis anterior and posterior	Tibia and fibula – posterior and anterior	Anterior base of 1st metatarsal. Posterior tarsals and metatarsals	Dorsiflexion, inversion and plantar flexion of foot
	Other muscles used in ankle and foot functions are: Fibularis longus and brevis, Hallucis longus flexor and extensor		

MUSCLES OF SCAPULA MOVEMENT

	ORIGIN	INSERTION	ACTION
Levator scapulae	Cervical vertebrae C1–C4	Scapula – superior medial border	Rotates scapula, lifts shoulder
Pectoralis minor	Clavicle, sternum	Humerus – bicipital groove	Flexes, adducts, medial rotates arm
Rhomboids major and minor	Thoracic vertebrae T1–T5 and cervical C7	Scapula – medial border	Adducts and rotates scapula
Serratus anterior	Upper nine costal cartilages (ribs)	Scapula – vertebral border	Rotates scapula, flexes shoulder
Trapezius	Occipital bone, cervical and thoracic vertebrae	Clavicle, scapula, acronium process	Lifts shoulder, adducts and rotates scapula

How muscles work

Muscles are made up of elongated cells called fibres that have a rich supply of blood vessels, lymph vessels and nerves. These components are encased in connective tissue called fascia, just as electrical cable has an outer casing with many different wires inside.

There are two different types of fibres: slow fibres, which contract slowly but keep going for a long time, and fast fibres, which contract quickly, but get tired rapidly. When a signal is received from the brain, the muscle cells become shorter and fatter as filaments within the cell slide against each other until they completely overlap. This causes the muscle as a whole to contract.

The fibres are organized in four configurations: parallel, circular, convergent and pennate (uni, bi or multi) depending on the direction and range of movement and strength required of the muscle.

Effects of massage on the muscles

Most massage work is related to the muscular system and the origins and insertion points of muscles. Tension produced in muscle is transmitted to the bones and joints via the connective tissue, and massage can address this tension and have beneficial effects.

Where injury occurs, followed by inflammation and healing, the connective tissue fibres and the fascia of adjacent muscle may stick together, creating an *adhesion*. This in turn can restrict range of movement and sometimes affect the nerves and blood supply to the muscle. Massage and passive stretching can help prevent adhesions forming and reduce complications. Muscle tone can be improved with massage and a host of muscle-related problems, the most common of which are listed below.

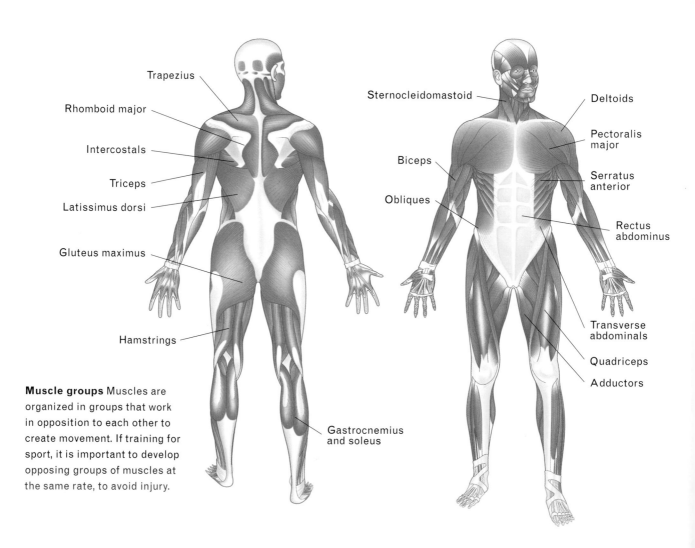

Trapezius
Rhomboid major
Intercostals
Triceps
Latissimus dorsi
Gluteus maximus
Hamstrings
Gastrocnemius and soleus

Sternocleidomastoid
Deltoids
Pectoralis major
Biceps
Serratus anterior
Obliques
Rectus abdominus
Transverse abdominals
Quadriceps
Adductors

Muscle groups Muscles are organized in groups that work in opposition to each other to create movement. If training for sport, it is important to develop opposing groups of muscles at the same rate, to avoid injury.

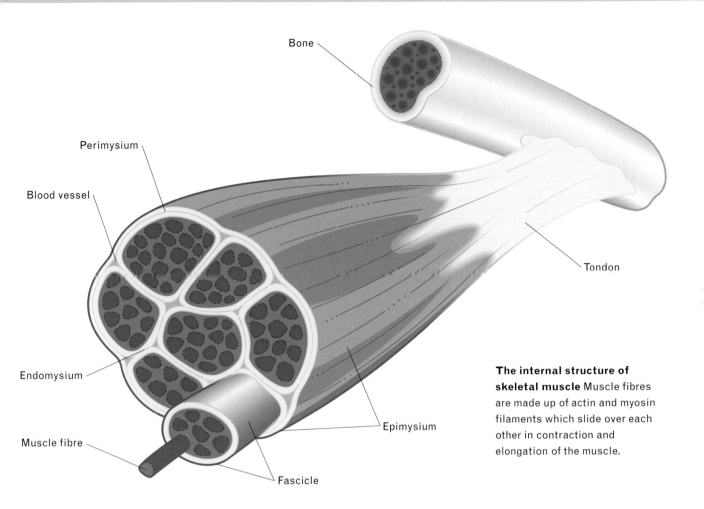

Bone

Perimysium

Blood vessel

Endomysium

Muscle fibre

Fascicle

Tondon

Epimysium

The internal structure of skeletal muscle Muscle fibres are made up of actin and myosin filaments which slide over each other in contraction and elongation of the muscle.

Massage for common conditions of the muscles

Atrophy
Muscle atrophy occurs when there is a marked decrease in the size of muscle as a result of lack of use or poor nutrition. More seriously, the wasting away of muscle also occurs with motor neurone disorder or muscular dystrophy.

Massage: Slow soothing strokes may increase range by mechanically broadening and stretching the tissue. Where muscle wasting is visible, the use of tapotement such as cross-fibre hacking, together with vibrational techniques, activates muscle spindles. They, in turn, stimulate contractions, helping to tone weak muscles.

Fibromyalgia
Often referred to as fibrositis, this is the inflammation of muscle and connective tissue. The condition results in pain and stiffness and often develops after infection,

trauma and even changes in weather. The symptoms are similar to more serious conditions such as lupus, so tests by a physician are recommended to establish the correct diagnosis.

Massage: Slow, gentle strokes such as effleurage, feathering and rocking will promote muscle relaxation.

Repetitive strain injury
See page 220.

Shin splints
See page 228.

Spasm
Stress, usually caused by injury or excess tension, can result in a localized contraction often referred to as a 'knot' or rigid area of muscle. This causes excessive motor nerve activity known as a muscle spasm, which cannot be relaxed voluntarily.

Massage: Once you have determined the spasm is from injury and not from another source, use effleurage to increase circulation, bringing fresh blood into the area. When the area is warm, apply friction techniques and passive stretching to lengthen the muscle and separate the fibres.

Spasticity

A muscle that resists stretch is usually described as spastic or hypertonic. This condition typically affects the arm flexors and leg extenders and can be recognized by the increase in muscle tone and reflexes, together with stiffness. Spasticity can range in form from very mild, for example as a result of a sports injury, to severe in the case of individuals with spinal cord injury or post stroke, where there may also be neurological repercussions.

Massage: Effleurage will increase circulation to the areas and help prevent adhesions forming. For sports injuries, venous and lymphatic massage are applied to reduce any oedema and following effleurage, kneading and petrissage strokes are used to ease tension and release the spasticity. If the symptoms are severe, massage should be applied with the knowledge of the client's physician and adjusted according to their impairments.

Strains

Forced stretching or a violent contraction can cause a strain injury to a muscle or tendon. These are very common in footballers. In a first-degree strain up to 10 per cent of the muscle or tendon is affected, resulting in only mild pain and swelling. A second-degree strain is

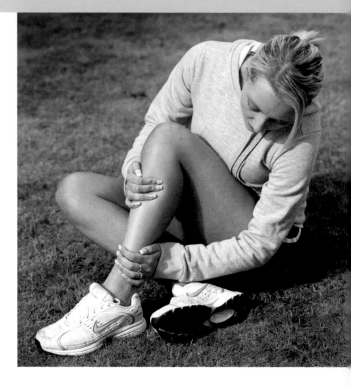

Sports injury A sudden violent muscle contraction can sometimes result in a strain injury, common to sports, in particular football and athletics.

where 10–99 per cent of the muscle or tendon is torn; in these cases the joint cannot cope with moderate resistance and movement is painful. There may also be oedema. In a third-degree strain 100 per cent of the fibres are torn and often a snap can be clearly heard at the time of injury.

Massage: Depending on the degree of strain, rest and ice should be applied for the first two to three days. Gradually introduce massage to maintain range of movement and prevent adhesions forming. Effleurage followed by some gentle friction work, icing the area before and after the treatment, can be effective. Slowly increase the treatment time as the healing allows.

Tendonitis

As the name suggests, this condition involves pain and swelling of the tendon. It is caused by trauma, overuse or a sudden action that pulls the muscle.

Massage: Treatment is very similar to that for a strain; resting and icing for the first two to three days before giving a massage.

OTHER TERMS IN MUSCLE PATHOLOGY

Other terms you may come across in pathology relating to muscles are:

- Cramp – a very mild form of spasticity sometimes caused by a salt deficiency.
- Sprain – a tearing of a ligament, categorized in degrees as for strains.
- Rupture – a tear in muscle fibres, tendons or fascia.
- Fatigue – a muscle finds it difficult to contract even with nerve stimulation.
- Tone – the level of tension in a resting muscle.

Digestion

Digestion has two separate processes: the passage of food through the body and the chemical break down of the food in order to extract elements required to maintain the body. These processes occur in the digestive tract and its associated organs.

The digestive tract, or alimentary canal as it is known, is an amazing 9m (30ft) from mouth to anus. Using powerful muscles along its length, it forces the food along by tonic and rhythmic contractions in a motion called peristalsis.

The digestive process takes place in four stages: *ingestion*, which is the taking in and swallowing of food, followed by *digestion*, where the food is broken down, *absorption*, which is the transfer of food through the wall of the intestine to the circulatory system, and finally *elimination*, in which the end products of digestion (i.e. undigested or unabsorbed food) are removed from the body.

All the main organs of the digestive system have specific functions in ingesting and extracting the components from food and drink as it passes through the digestive tract. The mouth is the first stop in the journey; the teeth chew the food to break it up, and the three salivary glands in the mouth secrete enzyme-containing saliva to begin the digestive process.

Once the food has travelled down the throat it enters the oesophagus, which is a muscular tube linking the pharynx to the stomach. It can take up to to 2–3 hours for a carbohydrate meal to be broken down and leave the stomach.

The next stop on the digestive journey is the small intestine. This is lined by small, finger-like projections called villi containing blood and lymph capillaries and is the location for most of the digestive process, separating out the nutrients and sending them off to the liver and transforming carbohydrates into simple sugars. The small intestine consists of three parts and in total is an incredible 5–6m (17ft) long. The duodenum is the top part; this is where pancreatic juice is added to break down protein. The jejunum is the middle part, followed by the ileum that leads to the large intestine; both continue to neutralize and absorb food as it passes through.

The large intestine, also known as the colon, has no villi and does not produce digestive enzymes. Instead it

SENSE OF TASTE

Whilst food is held in the mouth at the start of the digestive process, over 100,000 taste buds located on the tongue send messages to the brain about the molecules of the food they have contact with. These messages help the body respond and determine if the matter is edible and whether it is sweet, sour, salty, etc. It will also provoke a emotional response related to whether it is likeable or not.

eliminates waste from the digestive tract via the anal canal. The large intestine is 1.5m (5ft) long and is so called because its diameter is much greater than that of the small intestine. The 'S' shaped end of the colon contains the rectum and anal canal. By the time it reaches this point, all that is left of ingested food is water and undigested matter and bacteria. The water is absorbed and returned to the blood and the remainder, or faeces, continue the final stage of the journey aided by peristalsis. Waste can take from one to three days to journey through the large intestine before being expelled through the anus.

The accessory glands

The chemical process of breaking down the food matter and utilizing the nutrients extracted involves the accessory glands of the digestive system, which are the salivary glands, the pancreas, gall bladder and liver.

Saliva in the mouth begins the digestive process. Three pairs of salivary glands produce enzyme-containing saliva: the parotid, below and in front of the ear; the

The pancreas This gland is composed of cell clusters (acini) that secrete pancreatic juice containing a number of enzymes concerned in digestion. It also has an important role in the endocrine system, producing hormones such as insulin.

The liver A great detoxifier, the liver is particularly important in the digestive process. Harmful toxins that are not water-soluble are combined in the liver with natural enzymes, so they become water-soluble and can be passed to the kidneys or bowel for excretion.

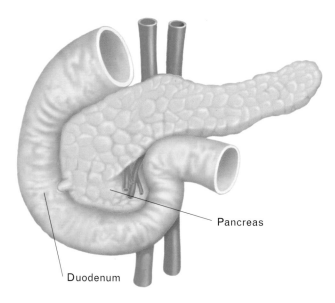

Pancreas

Duodenum

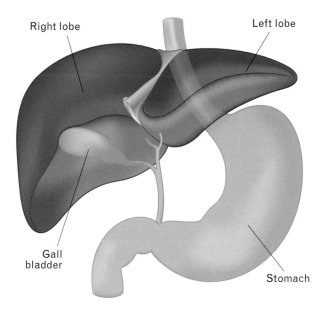

Right lobe

Left lobe

Gall bladder

Stomach

submandibular, below the jaw, and the sublingual, under the tongue. Saliva helps to moisten and soften the food, whilst the enzymes start the break down of starch to sugar.

The pancreas is positioned behind the the stomach and is both an exocrine gland, secreting a digestive enzyme known as pancreatic juice which reduces acid in the stomach, and an endocrine gland secreting the insulin and glucagon hormones to regulate sugar in the blood. The pancreatic juice passes to the duodenum to help break down proteins.

The gall bladder, located in a depression on the surface of the liver, is a pear-shaped sac that stores the bile secreted from the liver before its controlled release into the duodenum.

The liver is the body's largest gland and, after the skin, the largest organ. It is located to the right of the stomach, under the diaphragm and has three important functions:

- **Production**: The liver secretes bile that emulsifies fats and because this is a continuous process, excess is stored in the gall bladder for use when required. Heat and energy are also produced, as well as heparin

which is important in preventing blood clotting in the blood vessels. A by-product of the liver's protein absorption process is uric acid.
- **Storage**: The liver stores glycogen, iron and vitamins A, D and B until needed. The iron is obtained from the break down of worn out red blood cells.
- **Metabolism**: The liver manufactures plasma proteins, detoxifies drugs and poisons including alcohol and plays an important part in the metabolism of proteins, fats and carbohydrates. Proteins are converted into usable carbohydrate, fats are desaturated and oxidized and excess carbohydrates converted to fat for storage.

Effects of massage on digestion

A well-balanced diet is necessary for the maintenance of good health and consists of the correct levels of proteins, carbohydrates, fats (lipids), mineral salts, vitamins and water.

Massage can help digestion and hence nutrition by helping the removal of waste products and increasing blood and lymph circulation. This in turn creates a demand for an increased supply of nutrients, which may bring about an improvement in appetite.

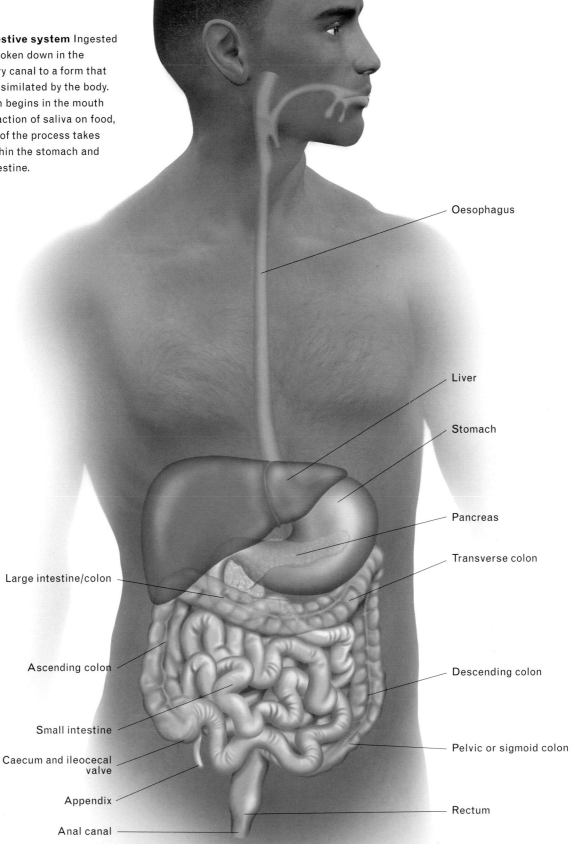

The digestive system Ingested food is broken down in the alimentary canal to a form that can be assimilated by the body. Digestion begins in the mouth with the action of saliva on food, but most of the process takes place within the stomach and small intestine.

Oesophagus

Liver

Stomach

Pancreas

Transverse colon

Large intestine/colon

Ascending colon

Descending colon

Small intestine

Caecum and ileocecal valve

Pelvic or sigmoid colon

Appendix

Rectum

Anal canal

CASE STUDY **DIGESTIVE**

CLIENT PROFILE

Maureen is a 32-year-old executive whose job takes her constantly away from home during the week. Her eating patterns are irregular and often she grabs a bite to eat late at night from a take-away or room service in the hotels that she stays at. Lately Maureen has found it difficult to pass stools and as a consequence also experiences abdominal pain, headaches and more flatulence than usual. The condition has begun to cause her embarrassment and discomfort. She mentioned this to a family friend who was a nutritionist and was told that it was her poor lifestyle and imbalanced diet that was causing the constipation, often the result of insufficient intake of natural fibre and fluids. She recommended a change in eating patterns and a visit to a massage therapist to stimulate her digestive system and get things moving.

REGULARITY

An initial treatment was followed up by weekly sessions until Maureen's constipation was eliminated and regular defaecation returned. Feeling the benefits of the massage treatments, Maureen continued to visit the massage therapist on a monthly basis and introduced extra sessions when work was intense and it was difficult for her to maintain a balanced lifestyle.

TYPE OF TREATMENT

The first treatment introduced gentle relaxation in order to expand the intestinal sphincters and promote movement of any contents. Deeper effleurage in a clockwise motion was applied over the ascending and descending colon, followed by some vibrational techniques. In further sessions percussive strokes were used around the sacral area in order to stimulate the digestive process.

OUTCOME

After the first massage session, Maureen felt some relief and a reduction in the constipation. She felt less bloated and the headaches and abdominal pain became less frequent. During the following weeks, together with more awareness of her poor lifestyle, her bowel movements were regulated and she had more energy and a healthier skin tone.

Abdominal massage promotes the production of digestive secretions through its reflex influence on glands and circulation of the stomach and intestines and so helps the absorption of food.

By stimulating peristaltic activity in the colon, the expulsion of waste is promoted, helping to relieve constipation and get rid of any intestinal gases.

Massage for common digestive conditions

Colitis

Colitis is inflammation of the inner layer of the colon. It is not known what causes this common condition, which manifests in weight loss, diarrhoea and bleeding. Ulceration may also be present and it can be very painful.

Massage: If pressure of touch causes pain, then massage is contraindicated. At other times, position the client so that they are comfortable, using pillows or bolsters where necessary, and apply gentle flat-handed effleurage to the abdomen, working in the direction of the intestine (clockwise) until the area is relaxed.

Constipation

Constipation is a common occurrence usually caused by poor diet. Lack of fibre and fluids in the diet combined with little physical activity makes the passing of stools infrequent and difficult and they remain in the bowel longer than necessary. Other physiological conditions such as pregnancy and diverticulitis can also result in constipation.

Massage: As with colitis, position the client comfortably, and working in a clockwise direction, circle the abdomen using gliding strokes either one or two handed. This may help movement by relaxing the lower digestive tract and promote the elimination process.

Crohn's disease

Crohn's disease is a chronic condition of unknown origin. It is a progressive inflammation of the digestive tract, usually affecting the ileum. It can often be confused with colitis because of its early symptoms of severe abdominal pain, diarrhoea and loss of appetite. However, high temperature and nausea may also be experienced. A person may suffer once or twice with the condition or experience bouts throughout life.

Massage: As with colitis, if the pressure of touch is painful, massage is contraindicated. At other times abdominal massage using effleurage in a clockwise direction is recommended to soothe the condition.

Diverticulitis

Diverticula are small pouches sticking out of the side of the colon. When these become inflamed the condition is called diverticulitis. This can cause severe pain and obstruction or even perforation of the bowel. The main symptom is the increase or decrease in constipation or diarrhoea.

Massage: If the pain or symptoms are severe, massage is contraindicated. At other times abdominal massage described for other conditions is appropriate.

Eating disorders

Eating disorders such as anorexia nervosa and bulimia have both physical and psychological elements. Anorexia is the avoidance of eating over a prolonged time, resulting in emaciation and lack of sleep. People with bulimia alternate between binge eating and self-induced vomiting or use of laxatives.

Massage: General massage is helpful for all cases to improve physiological processes, induce relaxation and help with the emotions.

Obesity

Obesity is when there is an abnormal amount of subcutaneous fat, resulting in a person carrying 30 per cent more weight than desirable for their frame.

Massage: Apply firm massage over the areas with large fat deposits, taking care to position the client comfortably, using drapes large enough to maintain modesty. If the client is very obese it may be more suitable to massage on the floor and where oedema is present, keep the legs slightly raised and apply lymphatic massage.

Gastritis

Gastritis is the inflammation of the stomach lining and takes two forms, acute and chronic. It can be caused by food indulgence, alcohol or smoking or even food poisoning. It may be a side-effect of medication or a bacteria or virus. Chronic gastritis can indicate something more serious. The main symptom is abdominal pain.

Massage: Massage is contraindicated for acute gastritis but suitable for chronic conditions unless the pressure of touch is painful. As with other digestive conditions, place the client in a comfortable position and apply abdominal massage in a clockwise direction.

Irritable bowel syndrome

Irritable bowel syndrome (IBS) is sometimes referred to as spastic colon. It occurs when peristalsis in the bowel is irregular, which results in swings between diarrhoea and constipation, causing discomfort and

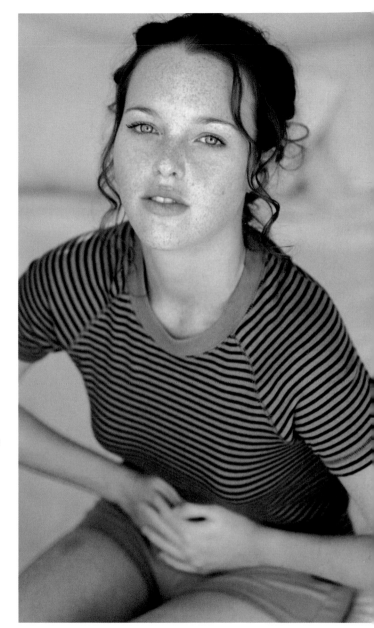

Digestive disorders These can be extremely debilitating. If the pressure of touch causes pain, in most cases, an alternative to massage is advisable.

bloating. It can be caused by emotional stress and is a very painful condition.

Massage: If the symptoms are not severe, massage can be helpful. As with other digestive conditions, position the client comfortably and apply general and abdominal massage. If the pressure of touch on the abdomen causes pain, avoid the area.

Circulation

The human body comprises 80 per cent fluid which needs to be moved and maintained by two systems collectively referred to as the circulatory system. They are known individually as the cardiovascular and lymphatic systems.

The circulation has seven major functions:

- It transports nutrients from the digestive tract to all parts of the body.
- It transports oxygen from the lungs to all parts of the body.
- It transports carbon dioxide and other wastes from cells to excretory organs such as the lungs, sweat glands of the skin and the urinary system.
- It transports hormones from the endocrine glands to various parts of the body.
- It helps to maintain body temperature.
- It helps to maintain fluid balance.
- It protects the body against disease.

The cardiovascular system

The cardiovascular system is made up of the heart and a network of blood vessels, through which blood is pumped by the heart to all parts of the body. The system is closed – that is, the blood stays within the network of veins, arteries and capillaries.

Blood is sometimes classified as a fluid connective tissue. It is made up of red blood cells (erythrocytes), which are bi-concave in shape to maximize their oxygen-carrying capacity, white blood cells (leukocytes), which form antibodies against disease, cell fragments (platelets), which are activated whenever blood clotting or repairs to blood vessels are necessary, filaments of fibrin, which enmesh red blood cells in clotting, and plasma, a straw-coloured liquid containing 90 per cent water and 10 per cent protein and other solutes.

Blood can be classified by the ABO system into types A, B, AB, and the commonest O. In the Rhesus system, blood is either positive or negative. Most Western Europeans are Rhesus positive and only 15 per cent of the population are the rarer Rhesus negative.

The average person has five to six litres of blood, which circulate every 60 seconds. Blood forms about 79 per cent of the body's weight and has three main functions: transport, regulation and protection.

Blood vessels

There are five types of blood vessel: arteries, arterioles, veins, venules and capillaries. All arteries carry rich, oxygenated blood to the cells of the body with the exception of the pulmonary arteries which carry de-oxygenated blood to the lungs for oxygenation. They are thick-walled, strong vessels that can expand to absorb the surge of blood resulting from each beat of the heart. The smallest arteries, called arterioles, branch into tiny vessels called capillaries. Their single-cell walls are so thin that they allow nutrients and oxygen to pass through into the surrounding tissues.

All veins carry blood that is low in oxygen, with the exception of the pulmonary veins, which return oxygenated blood from the lungs to the heart. Veins are thinner walled than arteries and have valves to prevent backflow of blood, especially in the legs. The smallest veins are called venules.

The heart

The heart is a hollow muscular organ that pumps blood around the body, supplying cells with oxygen and nutrients. It has four chambers: the left and right atria at the top and left and right ventricles at the bottom, with a muscular wall called a septum dividing it lengthways. The heart wall is made up of three layers: the endocardium (inner layer), the myocardium (middle layer and heart muscle) and the pericardium (outer layer or serous membrane).

Blood flow passes from the right to the left side of the heart via the lungs, hence the right side is low in oxygen and the left rich in oxygen. The right side flow is called pulmonary circulation and the left systemic circulation.

The blood enters the heart through the right atrium from the superior vena cava, then is pumped through the tricuspid valve into the right ventricle. When the right ventricle contracts, the blood is pushed into the pulmonary arteries which carry it to the lungs for oxygenation. The re-oxygenated blood enters the left atrium and passes through the mitral valve into the

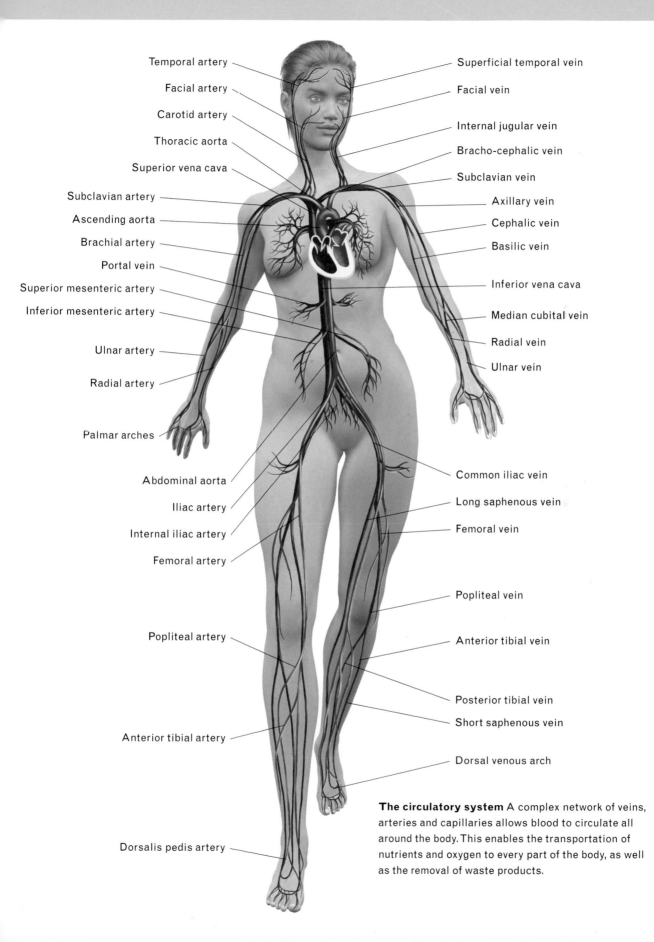

Temporal artery

Facial artery

Carotid artery

Thoracic aorta

Superior vena cava

Subclavian artery

Ascending aorta

Brachial artery

Portal vein

Superior mesenteric artery

Inferior mesenteric artery

Ulnar artery

Radial artery

Palmar arches

Abdominal aorta

Iliac artery

Internal iliac artery

Femoral artery

Popliteal artery

Anterior tibial artery

Dorsalis pedis artery

Superficial temporal vein

Facial vein

Internal jugular vein

Bracho-cephalic vein

Subclavian vein

Axillary vein

Cephalic vein

Basilic vein

Inferior vena cava

Median cubital vein

Radial vein

Ulnar vein

Common iliac vein

Long saphenous vein

Femoral vein

Popliteal vein

Anterior tibial vein

Posterior tibial vein

Short saphenous vein

Dorsal venous arch

The circulatory system A complex network of veins, arteries and capillaries allows blood to circulate all around the body. This enables the transportation of nutrients and oxygen to every part of the body, as well as the removal of waste products.

Blood flow through the heart

Oxygenated blood from the lungs arrives in the left atrium of the heart via two pulmonary veins, passing to the aorta and then on to the rest of the body. The venae cavae deposit de-oxygenated blood in the right atrium, from where it is pumped via the pulmonary artery to the lungs.

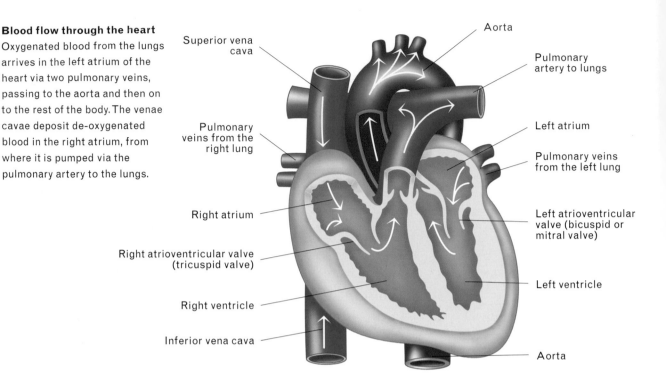

Superior vena cava

Pulmonary veins from the right lung

Right atrium

Right atrioventricular valve (tricuspid valve)

Right ventricle

Inferior vena cava

Aorta

Pulmonary artery to lungs

Left atrium

Pulmonary veins from the left lung

Left atrioventricular valve (bicuspid or mitral valve)

Left ventricle

Aorta

left ventricle from where it is pumped via the aorta to the body's circulatory system.

To achieve this pumping effect, the heart contracts and relaxes between each heartbeat. The heart chamber fills with blood during the relaxation or diastole period and expels the blood during the contraction or systole period. The terms diastolic and systolic are used in the measurement of the blood pressure against the arterial wall: a normal resting blood pressure measurement is 120 systolic over 80 diastolic.

The heartbeat is regulated by the autonomic nervous system. A resting or calm healthy heart beats 70 times a minute, but during stress, exercise or excitement this could rise as high as 200 beats a minute. The heartbeat can be measured by the pulse of an artery expanding and contracting.

The lymphatic system

The other half of the circulatory system, the lymphatic system, is the body's waste disposal unit, draining excess fluid from the tissues, absorbing fats from the intestine and returning them to the blood. At the same time it helps fight disease by producing lymphocytes. It consists of lymph, lymph vessels, lymphocytes and lymphatic organs.

Lymph or lymph fluid is the excess fluid from the tissues and intestine. In the absence of a pump, it flows by a series of one-way valves that move the fluid forward, aided by the activity of the skeletal muscles, pulsation of the neighbouring arteries and 'suction' from the respiratory system.

The lymph vessels, referred to as lymphatics, form a dense network reaching out to all the regions of the body. Smaller networks join together to form larger lymphatic vessels until they link with two collection points: the thoracic duct and the right lymphatic duct located in the chest cavity. These ducts eventually open into the blood vessels of the neck where lymph drains into the cardiovascular system. The largest lymph vessel is the thoracic duct, which runs up the front of the spine and empties into the left subclavian vein. The smaller, right lymphatic duct takes lymph from the upper right area of the torso and empties into the right subclavian vein.

At various points along the system the lymph passes through small, bean-shaped structures called lymph nodes that acts as filters, removing bacteria and large particles. Clusters of lymph nodes are found in certain areas of the body such as the armpits, groin, chest and abdomen. When the body is fighting an infection these lymph nodes commonly become swollen as the immune system is activated. The nodes swell from their regular 'pea' size to the size of marbles or larger, retracting after the infection.

Lymphatic organs

The two main organs of the lymphatic system are the thymus and the spleen, although there is also lymphoid tissue in the tonsils, appendix and intestines.

The thymus, which is also an endocrine gland (see page 73), is located in the neck, behind the sternum. It is a long flat organ that plays a key role in the body's immune system by secreting the hormone thymosin which stimulates the development of lymphocytes.

The spleen is located in the upper left area of the abdomen, behind the stomach. It serves as a reservoir for blood cells, being rich in blood vessels, and destroys old red blood cells and platelets. It also plays a part in the body's immune system and although it is possible to survive without a spleen, a person who has had their spleen removed will tend to be predisposed to infection.

The immune system

The human body has two main forms of defence against infection: non-specific (innate) and specific (adaptive). The non-specific defences include physical barriers such as skin and mucous membranes, and antibacterial secretions in the intestines. Specific defences occur in response to infection. When the body encounters a microorganism or molecule that it does not recognize it produces antibodies and then lymphocytes specific to the invader.

Some of the cells produced will remain in the body long after the infection has cleared up. These are memory cells that allow the immune system to recognize the pathogen if it occurs again. This ability, known as active immunity, is exploited in vaccination, in which memory cells are artificially stimulated by the introduction of an antigen derived from the organism to give a long-lasting defence against infection.

Passive immunity is short term and no memory cells are produced. It occurs when large quantities of antibodies are transferred from one individual to another, for example from a mother to her baby either in the womb or via breast milk.

Lymphocytes

The cells of the specific immune system are specialized white blood cells called lymphocytes. There are two main types: T and B lymphocytes.

T lymphocytes are produced initially in the bone marrow but then move to the thymus gland (hence 'T' cells), where they mature into various subtypes, such as helper T cells, memory T cells or cytotoxic T cells. They play a role in the cell-mediated immune response, in which cells called macrophages engulf and then digest cellular debris and pathogens.

CASE STUDY **CIRCULATION**

CLIENT PROFILE

Michael had recently been involved in a minor car crash. He received a gash to the head and was given hospital treatment before returning home. A week or so later he was still feeling unwell and suffered headaches, felt constantly tired but could not sleep and his skin tone was very pale. He went to see the company nurse at his work who diagnosed anaemia. The loss of blood at the time of the car crash had left him with a deficiency of haemoglobin or reduction of red blood cells. Iron tablets were prescribed, along with massage to increase circulation and enhance blood supply, which in turn promotes the production of red blood cells.

REGULARITY

A quick measure to remedy the situation was a course of daily massage sessions, each one short in duration, over a period of a week.

TREATMENT

General full body massage was applied using light pressure, to promote relaxation, rest and the circulatory systems. After day two, abdominal massage was introduced to improve the absorption of iron and vitamin B12, vital for the reduction of the condition.

OUTCOME

After a week of short treatments, together with the introduction of iron through medication, Michael's skin tone looked normal, he had started to sleep through the night and his stamina was slowly returning.

B lymphocytes, which are also produced in the bone marrow, are central to the humoral immune response. Antibodies produced by the B lymphocytes bind to antigens on the surface of invading microbes and identify them for destruction.

Effects of massage on the circulation

All massage movements improve and accelerate blood and lymph flow. Effleurage in particular assists venous and lymphatic return. Venous blood and lymph flows in one direction towards the heart and massaging in the same direction can mechanically assist this process.

Wringing and kneading strokes cause a temporary change in shape of the muscles, which in turn pressurizes the surrounding blood vessels, also resulting in the acceleration of venous return and speeding up the removal of toxins that can cause muscle aches and pains. Oxygenation, food delivery and waste disposal can all be accelerated with the application of massage.

Massage plays an important and effective role in relation to the lymphatic system. By applying specific techniques classified as manual lymphatic drainage, the movement of lymph and the reduction of fluid retention (oedema) can be achieved. It is necessary for the massage therapist to have knowledge of the route and direction that lymph drainage takes in order to apply the strokes, particularly when used in a clinical setting. Sometimes in the treatment of breast cancer, the lymph nodes are removed or damaged, causing interference to the natural drainage process of the upper limb. The oedema that occurs can be dispersed manually with massage until new lymphatic vessels grow back.

Massage for common circulatory conditions

Anaemia

Anaemia is a condition where the blood is not able to supply the body with an adequate supply of oxygen. Translated as 'without blood', anaemia can be caused by lack of iron or the loss of large amounts of blood and is often an indication of other physiological problems. It sometimes occurs during pregnancy, particularly if the mother is vegetarian, which can result in iron deficiency. Some of the signs of anaemia are tiredness, pale skin colouring, headaches and a tendency to feel the cold.

Massage: For mild anaemia adjust the style and duration of the massage to the client's energy levels: slow and gentle when fatigued, more dynamic and a longer session when more energized. Where the condition is due to blood loss, apply the strokes using very light pressure to encourage venous flow.

Aneurysm

An aneurysm is a weakened area in the wall of a blood vessel that bulges outwards. Usually located in the aorta or base of the brain, aneurysms are more common in people with high blood pressure. If not treated they can grow in size until they burst with fatal consequences.

Massage: It is advisable for the client to obtain consent from their physician before receiving massage. In the case of an abdominal aortic aneurysm do not massage the abdomen or psoas. General massage will help reduce high blood pressure, in particular the use of long sweeping strokes.

Angina

Angina is a pain that occurs when the heart muscle is not receiving enough oxygen due to narrowing of the arteries that carry the blood supply to the muscle. The pain originates in the chest and travels down the left arm and it can be triggered by physical exertion, emotional stress or exposure to intense cold, in fact any circumstance where there is a need for extra oxygen supply. It can also be a warning that there is heart disease present.

Massage: General relaxation promoted by a full body massage is useful for a client who has had an angina attack. Received on a regular basis massage may help prevent any further occurrences. Make sure that the treatment room is warm and the client well draped and do not use hot or cold packs as part of the massage. If a client has an angina attack during a massage treatment, place them in the seated recovery position and check if they have any medication with them to take. Get assistance if necessary.

Hypertension or high blood pressure

Hypertension or high blood pressure is a common condition in today's world. Normal blood pressure readings which relate to the pressure blood asserts on the walls of the heart and arteries is 120/80 systolic over diastolic pressure. High blood pressure is defined as sustained pressure of 140/90 or above. Over time, if the hypertension is constant, the arterial walls become rigid and resist the flow of blood, which can lead to heart disease or a stroke. Long-term hypertension is often the result of poor lifestyle conditions, lack of exercise, obesity and smoking, but it can also be inherited. Short-term hypertension can be the result of an adrenaline rush or moments of stress that cause the heart rate to rise. This will pass once the situation is over and the blood pressure rate will return to normal.

Massage: Deep relaxation routines using long gliding strokes can promote relaxation and, combined with changes in lifestyle, help to reduce the blood pressure. During a regular treatment, blood pressure tends to go down which is why the client should be advised to get up slowly from the table in case they feel momentarily light headed. Massage is not a substitute for medication in high risk conditions but can be very effective in moderate cases.

Raynaud's syndrome

See page 222.

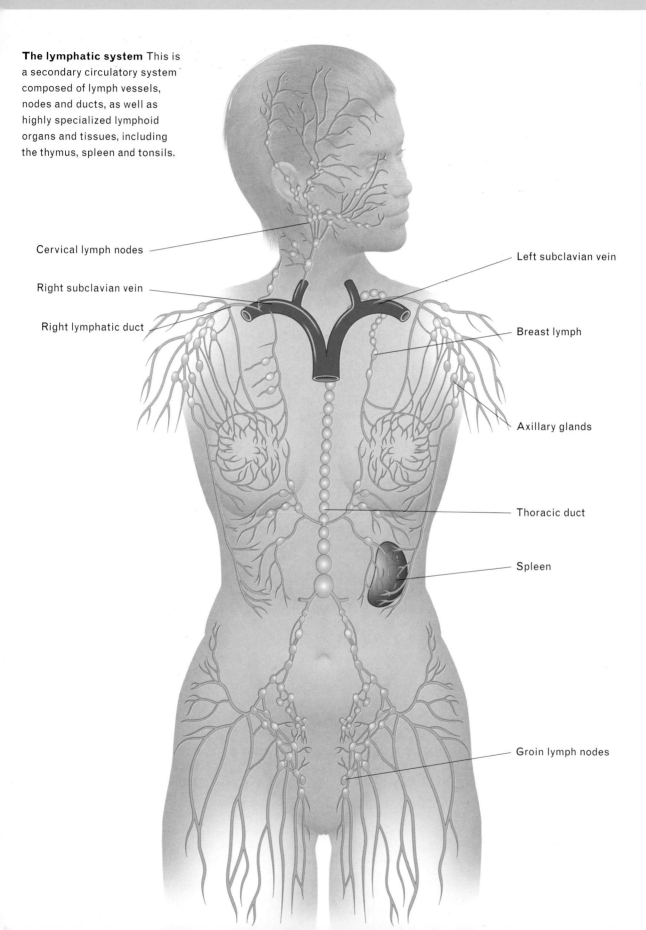

The lymphatic system This is a secondary circulatory system composed of lymph vessels, nodes and ducts, as well as highly specialized lymphoid organs and tissues, including the thymus, spleen and tonsils.

Cervical lymph nodes

Right subclavian vein

Right lymphatic duct

Left subclavian vein

Breast lymph

Axillary glands

Thoracic duct

Spleen

Groin lymph nodes

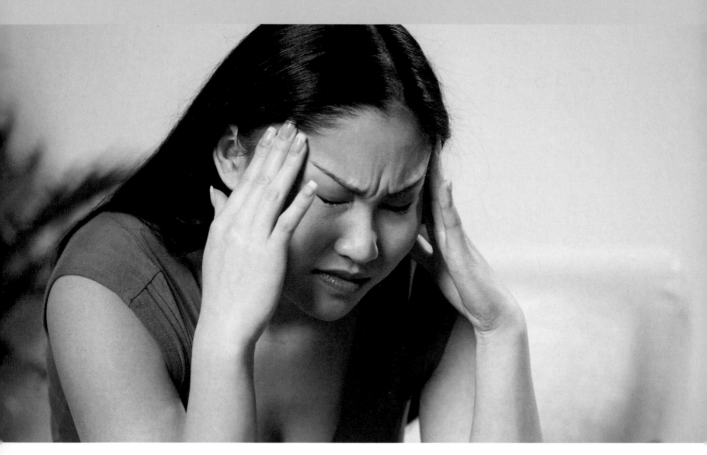

Migraine The clinical signs and symptoms of migraine headaches point to a disrupted regulation of the circulatory system.

Sickle cell disease

Sickle cell disease is an inherited form of anaemia caused by abnormal haemoglobin. The red blood cells are formed in the shape of a sickle hence the name. Because of the shape less oxygen can be supplied to the body tissues which in the long term can result in tissue damage. There is no cure for this disease and it can be extremely painful. Its other symptoms are lethargy, headaches and thrombosis.

Massage: It is advisable to get the client to obtain approval for massage from their physician before treating and not to treat during any flare ups. Otherwise apply general massage, adjusting your technique and pressure to the client's stamina levels. Take extra post-treatment care, assisting them when required to do so.

Varicose veins

These are enlarged and lumpy veins that occur where the valves have collapsed, preventing blood flowing at a normal rate. This in turn overloads the vein and the walls push outwards and become overstretched. Varicose veins are usually found in the lower limbs and can be painful and swollen. The condition often arises during pregnancy, or in people who are required to stand for long periods in their employment. Crossing the legs or wearing constricting clothing over the area exacerbates the problem.

Massage: Over and below the area, massage is contraindicated so as not to encourage more blood into the constricted veins. However it is safe to massage from above the localized area and continue the massage as normal. The client may find it comfortable to have the legs slightly elevated during the massage.

Migraine

Vascular headaches, including migraines and cluster headaches, occur due to dilation of the blood vessels in the head. They often result in nausea, vomiting and fatigue and are followed by a need for sleep. Migraines can be triggered by foods such as cheese, chocolate or red wine. Hormone changes during pregnancy and menopause can also cause regular suffering. Cluster headaches are similar to migraines but occur one after the other over a period of several days.

Massage: Treatment is contraindicated during the migraine or cluster headache but between attacks general massage is recommended and may even help reduce the frequency of headaches as the body learns to relax.

Nervous system

The nervous system, consisting of the brain and spinal cord, as well as sensory and motor nerves throughout the body, works closely with the endocrine system to maintain homeostasis.

A highly complex system, made up of billions of nerve cells called neurons and their supporting connective tissue (neuroglia), the nervous system is split into two parts known as the central nervous system (CNS) and the peripheral nervous system (PNS).

The functions of the nervous system are:

- Reception – receiving messages.
- Transmission – delivering to the CNS by sensory (afferent) nerves.
- Integration – interpreting messages.
- Transmission – transmitting messages by motor (efferent) nerves.
- Response – messages sent to the body.

The CNS interprets incoming sensory information and sends out instructions in the form of motor responses. It is the control centre for thoughts and emotions.

The PNS can be subdivided into the somatic nervous system, which carries information to the brain from all the senses and the musculoskeletal system in a controlled or voluntary way, and the autonomic nervous system, which sends uncontrolled or involuntary impulses from the heart, glands and smooth muscle via sympathetic and parasympathetic pathways.

The CNS comprises the brain, meninges, spinal cord and cerebrospinal fluid.

The brain

The brain is one of the body's largest organs, containing billions of neurons which use glucose as their energy source. As glucose cannot be stored, a continuous supply of oxygen from the respiratory system is needed to break it down, which is why deprivation of oxygen kills brain cells in minutes.

Divided into two large cerebral hemispheres, the four main parts to the brain are the brainstem, cerebrum, diencephalon and cerebellum.

The brainstem connects the cerebrum and cerebellum to the spinal cord and has three parts, the medulla, pons and midbrain. The medulla contains the vital cardiac, respiratory and vasomotor (blood pressure) centres. Motor fibres conduct the impulses between the brain and spinal cord in a crossover pathway – the left side of the brain controlling the right side of the body and vice versa. The pons acts as the bridge to other parts of the brain and also regulates respiration. The midbrain controls the visual and auditory centres and movements that wake the body from sleep and maintain consciousness.

The cerebrum is the centre for intellect, memory, thought, language and emotion. It is the largest section of the human brain and is divided into two hemispheres, right and left. It has two layers, the outer cortex or grey matter and the inner layer or white matter. White matter also has six lobes, each with a specific functions relating to sensory, motor and association (intellectual) activities.

The diencephalon is located between the cerebrum and midbrain and contains the thalamus, a major relay centre that transmits sensory information (except smell) to the cerebrum, and the hypothalamus, the centre that regulates mechanisms essential to homeostasis such as body temperature, water balance, endocrine control and the link between the endocrine and nervous systems.

The cerebellum is responsible for coordination and balance. It also consists of two hemispheres filled mostly with white matter encased in an outer layer of grey matter.

The meninges

The meninges are the three layers of connective tissue that cover the brain and the spinal cord. The tough outer layer is the dura mater, the second layer is a thin, delicate membrane known as the arachnoid, and the third inner layer is a very thin membrane with many blood vessels called the pia mater.

The spinal cord

The spinal cord is a slightly flattened cylinder composed of grey and white matter that runs in the vertebral canal of the spine, extending from the brain to the lumbar region. Its function is to control reflexes and transmit information back and forth from the PNS to the brain through ascending and descending pathways.

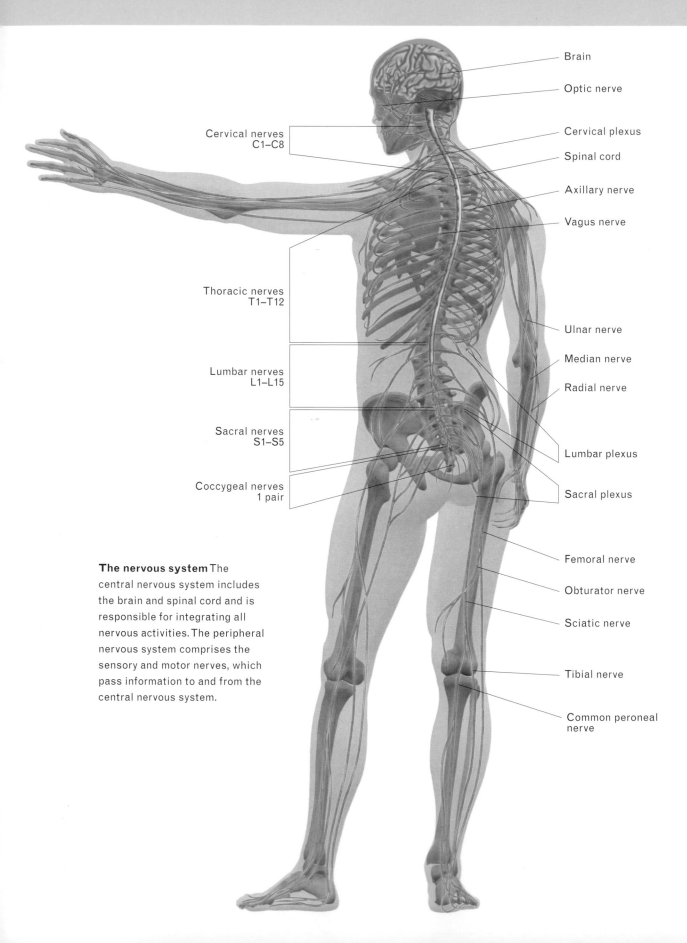

Brain

Optic nerve

Cervical nerves
C1–C8

Cervical plexus

Spinal cord

Axillary nerve

Vagus nerve

Thoracic nerves
T1–T12

Ulnar nerve

Median nerve

Lumbar nerves
L1–L15

Radial nerve

Sacral nerves
S1–S5

Lumbar plexus

Coccygeal nerves
1 pair

Sacral plexus

Femoral nerve

Obturator nerve

Sciatic nerve

Tibial nerve

Common peroneal
nerve

The nervous system The central nervous system includes the brain and spinal cord and is responsible for integrating all nervous activities. The peripheral nervous system comprises the sensory and motor nerves, which pass information to and from the central nervous system.

Cerebrospinal fluid

Cerebrospinal fluid (CSF) acts as a shock absorber, protecting the brain from injury. It is a clear fluid made of water, mineral salts, glucose and proteins, and circulates through the ventricles (cavities) and spaces of the brain and spinal cord, providing nourishment and protection.

Sampling of the CSF by lumbar puncture and pressure measurements can be used in the diagnosis of diseases such as meningitis and multiple sclerosis.

The peripheral nervous system

The peripheral nervous system is made up of 12 pairs of cranial nerves linking the brain with sensory receptors and muscles and 31 pairs of spinal nerves linking the spinal cord with various structures.

There are two types of nerve fibres: *dendrites* that receive neural messages and *axons* that transmit neural messages from cell bodies to other neurons, muscles or glands. A nerve is a bundle of axons wrapped in connective tissue and each nerve cell has only one axon. The cells or neurons of the PNS are specialized to receive and transmit messages or neural impulses and have their own protective glial cells.

Effects of massage on the nervous system

The nervous system is in close alliance with the skin, blood and muscular systems and so massage of all of these areas will produce a response in the nerves. Various massage procedures produce an effect upon the nervous system through the influence of manipulation upon nerve endings.

Massage for common conditions of the nervous system

Alzheimer's disease

This is a form of dementia characterized by memory failure, confusion and disorientation. It affects the cognitive functions that control the personality and language. The disease affects the memory first, gradually worsening over time.

Massage: Focus on techniques to maintain mobility, working on stiff joints and any areas of muscle tension. You will have to work with the client on their tolerances of time and pressure but do not exceed a regular full body treatment time of 90 minutes.

Bell's palsy

This is a condition where paralysis of one side of the face suddenly occurs due to the inflammation of a nerve (CN7). It may be a transient state lasting a few months or could be a permament condition. It is not really established what causes this to happen but it may be the result of some viral infection or trauma to the nerve. The palsy may also have an effect on the control of the eye and saliva on the paralysed side.

Massage: Include the face in the general massage using strokes to stimulate the muscles. Work in an upwards direction keeping the pressure light.

Bipolar and anxiety disorders

These disorders are becoming more commonplace. In bipolar disorder two phases – manic and depressive – tend to alternate, one phase becoming predominant at a time. Symptoms of the manic phase are limitless energy, hyperactivity and extremes of emotion and euphoria. The depressive phase manifests itself in reduced self-esteem, fatigue and deep feelings of guilt and sadness. The person may also feel chilled or flushed and these attacks can vary in frequence, usually lasting from a minute up to an hour at a time.

Massage: As a relaxant, massage can have beneficial effects for both types of disorder, but make sure that you have details of a contact or physician should a panic attack occur during a treatment.

Cerebal palsy

This is a congenital disorder causing damage to the motor area of the brain during the very early stages of life. It results in the loss of muscle control and coordination and sometimes impairs speech. The muscles may also be in spasm and a highly excited state. Cerebral palsy may be caused by problems during pregnancy such as rubella infection or malnutrition. The damage is irreversible but does not worsen.

Massage: If the cerebal palsy is severe it is advisable to obtain clearance from the client's physician before treating. Make sure that muscles are not forced into stretches and position the client's body carefully to give maximum comfort.

Multiple sclerosis

Often referred to as MS, this condition affects the central nervous system and is degenerative. The progressive destruction of the myelin sheaths around the nerves often begins in young adulthood and has periods where the condition worsens followed by remission before flaring up again. The symptoms range from light to severe according to the location of the damaged tissue but can include impaired speech or mobility.

Massage: Treatment is contraindicated during a flare-up, otherwise it is very beneficial in decreasing muscle rigidity and stiffness. The use of hot and cold packs is contraindicated at all times, and the duration and pressure should be adjusted to the client's stamina level.

Nerve impingement

This is something that you may come across frequently as a massage practitioner. It is caused by pressure against a nerve by adjacent tissues such as muscle, tendons or ligaments. This causes tightness and loss of range and is usually caused by overuse or injury that compacts the two elements. Another form of nerve impingement is when the nerve passes through the muscle and gets pressurized internally through the tightening of the muscle. The symptoms of both types are the presence of sharp, radiating pain which can lead to numbness or a pins and needles sensation.

CASE STUDY **NERVOUS SYSTEM**

CLIENT PROFILE
Paul works as a tree surgeon and while working in a team making a group of storm-damaged trees safe, his lower right leg became caught. It was a slight accident and no bones were broken, only some initial pain and bruising. He could move the leg as before but noticed that he had some loss of sensation in the calf and foot. It was diagnosed that the pressure of the impact had caused some nerve impingement which was resulting in the loss of sensation. Physiotherapy and regular massage were recommended by his physician.

REGULARITY
It was suggested that Paul initially went twice a week for short, focused treatments until sensation and strength began to return.

TYPE OF TREATMENT
The techniques used for this type of condition are focused and deep working. Neuromuscular techniques applied over small areas of approximately 5 cm (2 in) with the pads of the thumbs can help release impinged nerves and restore their functions. Often a release is encountered and pressure eased immediately.

OUTCOME
After one week of neuromuscular work, Paul's leg had full sensation and he was able to return to work.

Massage: The treatment should be very focused, working on the deep tissue for a short period. Use massage to promote relaxation and reduce the tension in the muscle causing the impingement.

Parkinson's disease

This is a neurological condition caused by a malfunction of the neurotransmitters that control movement. It can occur at any age and is degenerative and irreversible. The symptoms are poor posture, rigidity and the lack of facial expression. The muscles alternately contract and relax, resulting in tremors of varying degrees.

Massage: If the condition is severe, seek recommendation from a physician before treating. Massage techniques to reduce rigidity in the muscles are very beneficial but do not force them or the joints into movement that is resisted. Relaxation techniques may also have a temporary effect on muscle tremors.

Sciatica

This is a common disorder where the sciatic nerve, the longest in the body stretching from head to toe, is irritated and becomes inflamed. This can be caused by overuse, injury such as whiplash, or heightened emotional stress. It may also be caused by impingement or nerve entrapment. Pain and tenderness is usually felt in the the lower back and leg regions, and motor functions may be affected in severe cases.

Massage: Manipulation can be beneficial but only if the cause has been determined by the physician as certain impingements may require medical attention. Causes such as a tightening of muscles can be helped by focused massage, to reduce any atrophy or oedema present.

Strokes

Known medically as cerebrovascular accidents, strokes are caused by a blockage in the cerebal blood vessels which results in damage to brain tissue. The symptoms are weakness of the muscles in varying degrees, speech abnormalities and changes in sensations. Some recovery is possible depending on the extent and location of the damage. A stroke can be mild, not requiring hospitalization, or severe and even fatal.

Massage: The use of deep pressure is contraindicated for massage and any joint mobilization should be done with utmost care. General techniques to prevent stiffness and reduce the spasticity of the muscles will help with any postural problems. As with other conditions of the nervous system, tailor the duration of the massage to the client's stamina levels.

Endocrine system

Unlike the nervous system, which responds rapidly to stimulus using nerve impulses to cause changes, the endocrine system works slowly, using hormones as messengers to cause physiological changes.

The glands of the endocrine system are the hypothalamus, pituitary, thyroid gland, pineal gland, parathyroid glands, thymus, adrenal glands, pancreas, testes and ovaries. These regulate the system by producing chemical messengers called hormones that boost the speed at which organs or glands work.

The hypothalamus

Hormones are produced in response to signals from an area of the brain called the hypothalamus, which acts in conjunction with the pituitary gland. The hypothalamus is the gland that links the nervous and endocrine systems. It is located just above the brainstem and is responsible for the regulation of body temperature, hunger, thirst and certain emotional states. The hormones it synthesizes and releases are called neurohormones and these act on the pituitary, causing it to secrete further hormones.

The pituitary gland

Located at the base of the brain, the small, pea-sized pituitary gland regulates the activity of most the other endocrine glands in the body. It produces three important hormones known as trophic hormones that act to increase production of other hormones. These are thyroid-stimulating hormone (TSH), adrenocorticotrophic hormone (ACTH) and gonadotrophic hormone. It also produces two non-tropic hormones: growth hormone and prolactin.

The thyroid gland

The thyroid is situated in the neck and is responsible for the regulation of growth and development. It extracts iodine from the blood and produces hormones such as thyroxine and calcitonin.

Effects of massage on the endocrine system

The endocrine system and stress levels are inextricably linked, so any relaxation provided by massage will tend to have an effect on hormone levels. Some endocrine glands, such as the adrenals, are known to be extremely responsive to our emotions, resulting in effects such as 'butterflies in the stomach', when adrenaline is released as a response to fear. Cortisol is another hormone released in times of stress; this can delibitate the immune system. Relaxation induced through massage will lower the production of these hormones and in turn help reduce stress.

Massage also increases the levels of the neurotransmitters dopamine and serotonin, which are believed to help reduce stress and depression.

Massage for common conditions of the endocrine system

Diabetes mellitus

In this disorder blood glucose levels become excessive due to a variety of causes. It is classified into two types: Type 1 is where not enough insulin is produced by the body due to the destruction of production cells in the pancreas. The shortfall has to be injected several times a day to maintain a safe blood sugar level. Type 2 (or maturity-onset diabetes) is more common. It is often a result of poor diet, high in carbohydrates, and can usually be controlled through diet and exercise. Long term, diabetes can lead to high blood pressure, poor circulation and sight impairment.

Massage: Make sure that if the client is taking insulin that medication is to hand, and that the treatment allows for food and water intake if required. It is useful to have some candy or high-sugar drink available in case of emergency. Injection sites are contraindicated for up to two weeks, so work around those areas avoiding percussive or vibrational strokes. Use light pressure and feedback any noticeable bruising or cracks in the skin so the client is aware of them.

Graves' disease

This is a disorder of the thyroid caused by an autoimmune reaction which results in the enlargement of the lymph nodes and thyroid. Particular to this condition is the noticeable protrusion of the eyeballs. Symptoms are fatigue, loss of appetite, anxiety and hand tremors.

Massage: The throat and neck areas should be avoided and any lymph node areas that appear to be enlarged. Massage techniques should be gentle and the pace and duration dependent on the client's stamina.

Goitre

This is the name given to an enlarged thyroid gland, which can be caused by infection, inflammation or low levels of iodine intake from food.

Massage: The neck and throat areas are contraindicated for massage and as for other conditions of the endocrine system, adjusted in pace and duration to the client's stamina at the time of treatment.

Hypoglycaemia

A drastic reduction in the level of blood glucose is known as hypoglycaemia. This can be due to a dysfunction of the pancreas, poor diet or, in the case of someone with diabetes, an overdose of prescribed insulin. The person will feel weak, light-headed, hungry and may even experience some disturbance to the eyesight. If left untreated a state of hypoglycaemia can lead to delirium, a coma and even be fatal.

Massage: Once the condition has been addressed, general massage is suitable, keeping the pressure gentle and the duration a little shorter than usual. Make sure you check with the client during the treatment as to their condition.

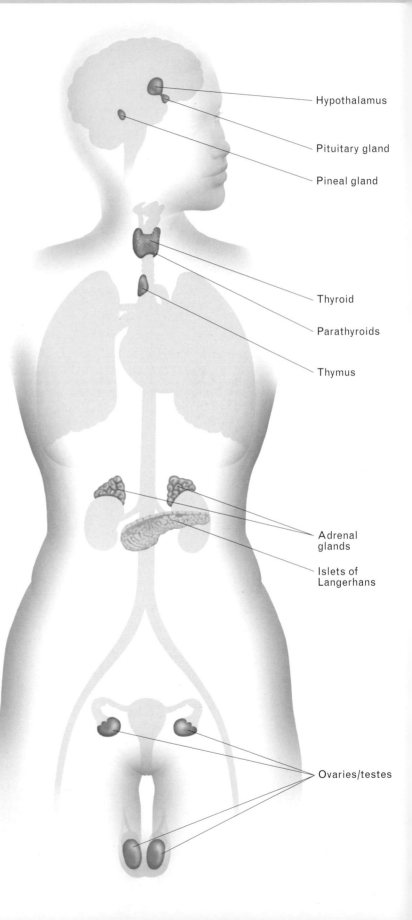

The endocrine system The endocrine glands and tissues produce hormones, the 'chemical messengers', and release them into the bloodstream. Endocrine glands and tissues include the pituitary, thyroid, parathyroid and adrenal glands, as well as the ovaries, the testes, part of the pancreas and the placenta.

Hypothalamus

Pituitary gland

Pineal gland

Thyroid

Parathyroids

Thymus

Adrenal glands

Islets of Langerhans

Ovaries/testes

ENDOCRINE GLANDS, THEIR LOCATION, RELATED HORMONES AND FUNCTIONS

GLAND	HORMONE	LOCATION	FUNCTION
Hypothalamus	Releasing and inhibiting hormones	Diencephalon of the brain	Stimulates and inhibits the secretion of other hormones
Pituitary			
anterior lobe	Thyroid-stimulating hormone (TSH)	Attached by a stalk to the hypothalamus in the brain	TSH acts on the thyroid gland
	Growth hormone (GH)		GH acts on the bones
	Adrenocorticotrophic hormone (ACTH)		ACTH acts on the adrenal cortex
	Gonadotrophins		Gonadrophins act on the testes and ovaries
	Prolactin		Prolactin acts on the mammary glands
posterior lobe	Antidiuretic hormone (ADH)	Attached by a stalk to the hypothalamus in the brain	ADH acts on the kidney tubules
	Oxytocin		Oxytocin acts on the mammary glands and uterine muscle
Thyroid	Thyroxine	Neck	Stimulates metabolism, growth and development
	Calcitonin		Lowers blood calcium
Parathyroid	Parathyroid hormone	On thyroid gland – bow shaped	Increases blood calcium levels and stimulates vitamin D
Pancreas *Islets of Langerhans (endocrine part of pancreas)*	Insulin and glucagon	Behind the stomach	Regulate blood sugar levels
Adrenal		Top of the kidneys	
Medulla (middle part)	Epinephrine (adrenaline) and norepinephrine (noradrenaline)		Help cope with short-term stress and effects and raise blood sugar
Cortex (outer part)	Cortisol and aldosterone		Help cope with long-term stress and raise blood sugar
Ovaries	Oestrogen and progesterone	Pelvis	Regulates development of sex characteristics and breasts Preparation of uterus for pregnancy
Testes	Testosterone	Pelvis	Regulates development of sex characteristics
Pineal	Melatonin	Below hypothalamus in brain	Controls puberty
Thymus	Thymosin	Chest	Immune functions

Reproductive system

The reproductive system ensures that the human species procreates and passes genetic material to offspring in order to sustain life. The structures and functions of the system develop and then operate in response to hormonal control.

CASE STUDY
REPRODUCTIVE AND URINARY

CLIENT PROFILE
June is 62 years old and has recently found it painful to pass urine. She began to worry about the condition when she noticed blood and the frequency and urgency to urinate increased. Her doctor diagnosed cystitis, a bladder infection that is common in females. She regularly visited a massage therapist and mentioned the condition on her next visit, unaware that the session could be tailored to promote the healing process.

REGULARITY
June's visits for massage were generally once a month but when she realized that it could help her condition she had two extra treatments that month.

TYPE OF TREATMENT
Light strokes similar to that of lymph massage were applied over the lower abdomen but avoiding any areas that were painful. Bladder problems can result in tension over the sacrum, the iliotibial tract and the areas above the pubic bone and the anterior thigh. These areas were addressed where touch did not cause discomfort.

OUTCOME
The massage together with medication cleared the condition up within three weeks and the passing of urine normalized.

The role of the reproductive system, in simple terms, is to ensure the combination of the male sperm and the female ovum or egg to form a new cell called a zygote. As the new cell divides it grows to form a new life – an embryo – which goes on to develop within the womb.

The male and female reproductive organs

The reproductive system is made up of ducts, cells and organs and their accessories, and the structure and function differs in males and females.

In the males, the system is made up of two testes, the seminal vesicle, the prostate gland, spermatic ducts and the penis.

The male sex cells or gametes are called spermatozoa. Produced by the testes in large quantities every day and stored in the seminal vesicles, the spermatozoa carry the genetic information from the male.

The female reproductive system comprises the ovaries, Fallopian tubes, uterus, vagina and accessory glands. Unlike the male system, in the female sex cells, or eggs (ova), are not produced continually in the ovaries – a woman is born with her lifetime quota and releases one egg roughly once a month from puberty to menopause.

Each sex cell or gamete only contains half the genetic information or genes required, so when the sperm fertilizes the egg to form a zygote this cell then contains 100 per cent of the chromosomes it requires, with genetic information from both parents.

Fertilization and implantation

The male testes contain tiny tubules which produce sperm that are stored until they are mature and able to swim. At this stage they enter a duct called the epididymis where they can stay up to four weeks before being expelled or reabsobed by the body. The seminal vesicle produces fluid to transport the sperm onwards and nourish it; it has a capacity of 50–100 billion sperm cells per cubic centimetre, and this mix of 90 per cent fluid and 10 per cent sperm is known as semen.

The female reproductive system Once the egg has been released from an ovary, it is drawn into the Fallopian tube. Slight contractions of the tube and the movement of tiny cilia move the egg towards the uterus. It can survive in the Fallopian tube for 24 hours and, if it is not fertilized, it will be reabsorbed by the body.

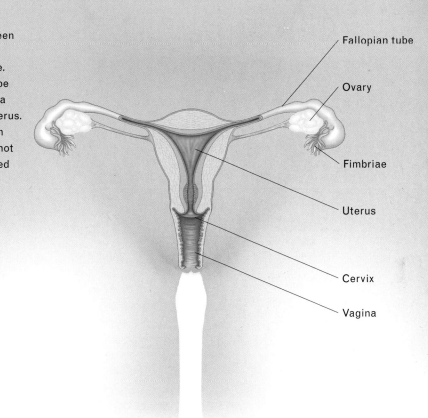

Fallopian tube

Ovary

Fimbriae

Uterus

Cervix

Vagina

To enable the sperm to merge with an egg, semen containing the sperm is ejaculated by the male penis into the female vagina, from where they attempt to reach the Fallopian tube and find eggs that have been previously released from the ovaries on maturity.

Following fertilization, in which the sperm and ovum merge together to form a zygote, the fertilized egg travels down the fallopian tube towards the uterus where it implants itself in the lining of the womb. At this stage it is referred to as an embryo. Placenta starts to form and the embryo is then connected to it via a duct called the umbilical cord through which nutrients and oxygen pass from mother to baby. Development is very fast from this point, the embryo becoming a foetus after eight weeks and remaining in the womb for a period of approximately 38 week from conception.

Birth

When the pregnancy ends the birth begins, starting with contractions followed by the delivery of the baby via the birth canal and finally the expulsion of the placenta.

During the pregnancy, the woman's body produces hormones called oestrogen and progesterone that prepare the mammary glands for feeding or lactation.

Menopause

A woman's productive life starts at first menstruation, when the mucous membrane lining the uterus is shed, a cycle that takes place every 28 days, until the age of approximately 45–55 years when the ovaries stop producing oestrogen and menstruation ceases. Known as menopause (see page 206), pregnancy usually becomes impossible after this 'change of life'.

Effects of massage on reproduction

Massage is thought to be able to help fertility in certain cases and in recent years programmes of massage and nutrition have shown excellent results. It is thought that massage can stimulate the production of hormones (testosterone in the man and relaxin in the woman) that help with sperm production and implantation of the fertilized egg respectively. This will increase the chances of pregnancy.

The male reproductive system
Male sperm production begins at puberty and continues until very late in life, although it starts to slow down in late middle age. Of the hundreds of million sperm in any one ejaculation, only a couple of thousand survive the journey into the uterus and on to the Fallopian tube.

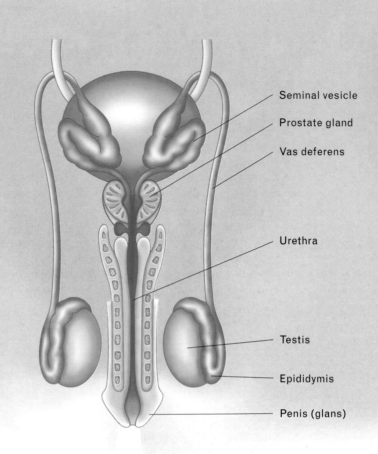

- Seminal vesicle
- Prostate gland
- Vas deferens
- Urethra
- Testis
- Epididymis
- Penis (glans)

Massage for common conditions of the reproductive system

Endometriosis
Endometriosis usually occurs in women between 20 and 40 years of age and who have not been pregnant. The condition occurs when the lining of the uterus develops in the pelvic cavity, abdomen or thorax and not in the uterus itself. Symptoms are painful menstruation and it can cause infertility.

Massage: General massage is beneficial, but ensure that the client is positioned comfortably. If there are emotional issues relating to infertility problems, referral to a specialist counsellor may be welcomed.

Ovarian cysts
Ovarian cysts are fluid-filled pouches that develop on the ovaries. They can grow quite large but are usually benign and have no effects on the physiological system and can be surgically removed. Symptoms are a swelling of the abdomen and some pain.

Massage: The abdominal area is contraindicated if painful to touch.

Mastitis
Mastitis is a condition of the mammary gland caused by a streptococcal infection that causes inflammation. It is most common during the first two months of breast feeding. Symptoms are pain, swelling and redness of the skin.

Massage: The upper chest area is contraindicated for massage and the positioning may have to be adapted for general massage if the condition does not allow the client to lie prone comfortably.

Sexually transmitted diseases
Sexually transmitted diseases, including genital herpes, syphilis, gonorrhoea and chlamydia are infections that are transmitted through sexual intercourse and through the placenta from mother to baby. Symptoms are usually inflammation, discharge and localized burning or itching. In severe cases they can result in infertility.

Massage: With all types of STD massage is contraindicated.

Respiratory system

Breathing is necessary for survival. The system through which the body takes in oxygen and expells carbon dioxide – the respiratory system – must work continuously without the need for conscious control for life to continue.

CASE STUDY **RESPIRATORY**

CLIENT PROFILE

Tom is a 19-year-old who suffers with asthma. It is affecting his studies and he feels self-conscious during attacks of breathlessness. These attacks are more regular during the summer months when pollen and dust are more prevalent. With exams coming up he asked his parents if there was anything he could do to reduce the symptoms. His mother sought the advice of her homeopath who suggested Tom had a course of massage treatments.

REGULARITY

For a month before his examinations, Tom visited a massage therapist every week for hourly treatments. On one occasion he had to postpone the treatment for a few days, due to an asthma attack brought on by a high pollen count in the atmosphere.

TYPE OF TREATMENT

One of the main benefits of massage for an asthmatic is relaxation, particularly in Tom's case with the stress of forthcoming examinations. General massage will promote the relaxation of the involuntary muscles of the respiratory tract and keep the airways open. Cupping strokes over the back area will help release any built-up mucus and friction over the intercostal muscles will improve local circulation.

OUTCOME

After three weeks of massage, Tom was more relaxed, his attacks were less frequent and intense, and his overall confidence had increased.

The process through which the body is supplied with oxygen and disposes of carbon dioxide is known as gas exchange and takes place in the lungs and their capillaries. Oxygen molecules from the air in clusters of tiny chambers called alveoli pass through the thin walls into the blood and are replaced with carbon dioxide. The final destination of the oxygen is the cells of the body where they are burned as fuel to produce energy in the form of ATP. The carbon dioxide or waste product is expelled.

Inhaled air comprises 20.9 per cent oxygen, 0.04 per cent carbon dioxide and 79 per cent nitrogen, whereas exhaled air is only 14 per cent oxygen compared to 5.6 per cent carbon dioxide and 79 per cent nitrogen. Without oxygen intake, the cells of the body would start to deteriorate in five minutes.

The respiratory system also plays a part in the smell and speech processes. Whilst inhaling, many scents enter the nasal cavities and stimulate nerve impulses that pass the information to the brain.

The movement of air over the vocal chords during respiration, combine together with the use of facial muscles and the tongue to produce speech.

The respiratory tract

The respiratory tract consists of two sections named the upper and lower tracts. The upper tract comprises the nose, nasal cavity, pharynx and larynx, whereas the lower tract is made up of the trachea, bronchi, alveoli, lungs and respiratory diaphragm.

Breathing begins with an intake of air through the nose into the nasal cavity, which is passed down through the pharynx and larynx into the trachea or windpipe as it is commonly known. Once there, air passes through a left and right bronchi to each lung. These bronchi are rather like tree roots that branch out into smaller passageways called bronchioles. These lead to alveoli which are tiny pockets within the lungs that participate in gas exchange. There are approximately 300 million alveoli in the lungs which, along with their capillaries, allow 900 millilitres of blood to engage in gas exchange.

The respiratory system

Oxygen is inhaled as air at the nose and mouth and taken to the lungs, where it is diffused through the alveoli walls into the blood cells. At the same time, carbon dioxide is absorbed from the blood into the alveoli, to be expelled through exhalation.

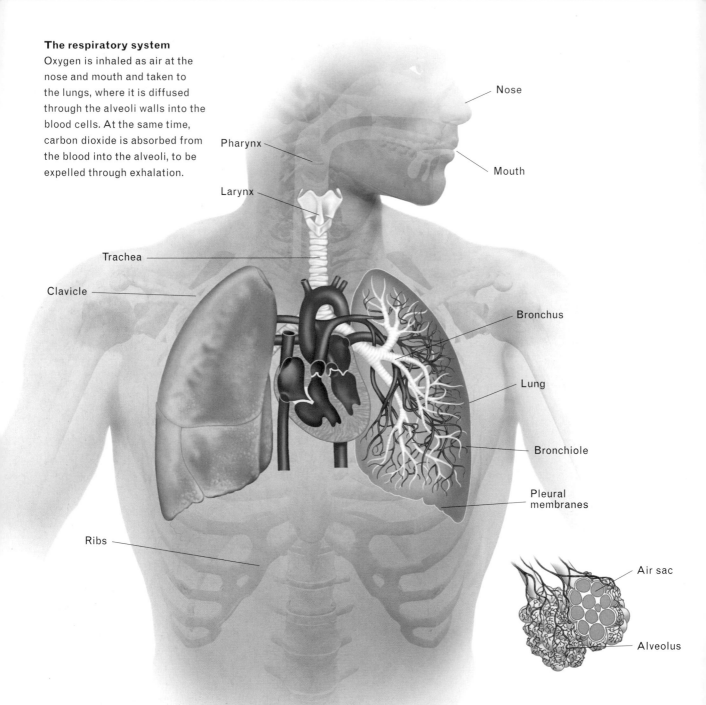

Nose

Mouth

Pharynx

Larynx

Trachea

Clavicle

Bronchus

Lung

Bronchiole

Pleural membranes

Ribs

Air sac

Alveolus

The main muscle used in the respiration process is the diaphragm. As you breathe in, the diaphragm contracts which in turn creates a vacuum in the chest cavity. This action sucks the air down into the lungs. On the out breath, the diaphragm relaxes, which in turn allows the lungs to deflate, expelling air through the mouth and nose.

During the respiration process a gaseous exchange takes place through the thin walls of the alveoli and blood capillaries that surround them. When inhaling, oxygen from the air enters the lungs and is collected in the alveoli where it is released into the bloodstream by diffusion through the blood capillary. The oxygen binds itself to the haemoglobin in the blood and is carried to cells around the body. At the same time, carbon dioxide is created as a waste product from these cells and is carried back to the lungs by the blood flow ready to be expelled through the wall of the alveoli and released on exhalation.

Effects of massage on respiration

The immediate and most visible effect that massage has is the slowing down of the respiration rate through relaxation. This will reduce any short or difficult breathing and, in the case of asthma, may be beneficial in reducing the frequency of attacks. Massage will help loosen tension in the respiratory muscles and fascia which in turn should increase capacity and volume and improve the respiratory flow.

For those using the larynx more than normal, such as singers or speakers, relaxation through massage will help reduce the extra tension stored in the muscles of the throat.

Where there is a build up of phlegm in the respiratory tract, specialized massage including tapotement techniques and positioning can loosen and drain the liquid away (see Chapter 8, page 204).

Massage for common conditions of the respiratory system

Asthma
See page 204.

Bronchitis

This is another inflammatory condition of the bronchi and can be an acute or chronic condition where the bronchial tubes swell and produce excess mucus. Acute bronchitis affects the upper respiratory tract, the symptoms being a high temperature and productive cough, whereas chronic bronchitis has symptoms of a prolonged productive cough and excessive mucus, smoking being its most common cause.

Massage: If the client has a temperature or is in a contagious stage, massage is contraindicated. To promote the drainage of congestion, percussive strokes applied to the back and costal areas with the client comfortably positioned is very effective. As for asthma, focus on the respiratory muscles.

Common cold and flu

These are two conditions affecting the respiratory tract. The common cold is a disorder of the mucosa of the upper tract, usually affecting the nose and throat and sometimes the larynx. It is a highly contagious viral disease spread by droplets and its symptoms include be sneezing and coughing, watering eyes, a sore throat or congestion, sometimes accompanied by a temperature or chill. If not addressed, this common disorder can develop into bronchitis or more serious respiratory conditions. Influenza, on the other hand, is an acute viral infection with a three-day incubation period. Its symptoms are an inflamed nasal mucosa, which can also be accompanied by muscle pain and headaches.

Massage: For the common cold, massage is contraindicated for the first 2–3 days after symptoms appear. Thereafter, provided the client is comfortable, general massage is suitable and working on the respiratory muscles may alleviate the symptoms. Massage is totally contraindicated for a client with influenza.

Emphysema

This disorder occurs when the air spaces in the lungs become enlarged and restrict exhalation and gaseous exchange. It is caused by the alveoli slowly being destroyed through overinflation. It is a chronic condition which can follow on from untreated bronchitis and is caused by irritation from pollution, industrial dust and cigarette smoking.

Massage: As with other respiratory conditions, focus the massage on the muscles of the respiratory system, adjusting the duration and pressure to the comfort level of the client.

Hayfever

This is a common condition and the general term for any allergic reaction of the nasal mucosa. Its symptoms are sneezing, itching and watery eyes and the cause could be a variety of things including dust, pet hair or pollution. In warm weather, high levels of pollen in the atmosphere can bring on this allergic reaction.

Massage: During a hayfever attack, massage is contraindicated. At other times refer to the case history and ensure that any allergens that could cause problems are avoided in the treatment area. Avoid positioning the client in a prone position or using a face cradle as this may exacerbate any nasal congestion.

Pleurisy

This is an extremely debilitating condition caused by inflammation of the pleural membranes. Breathing becomes very painful as the swollen membranes rub against each other and a chronic condition can lead to permanent adhesions.

Massage: It may be advisable for your client to obtain clearance from their physician, even though pleurisy is not contraindicated for massage. Focus on the respiratory muscles and take into account the physical stamina of the client.

Skin

Also known as the integumentary system, the skin is the largest organ of the body. It covers the whole musculoskeletal frame in various degrees of thickness and its tone reflects our physiology. A client's appearance will tell us a lot about their lifestyle and condition.

The skin is made up of two layers: the epidermis and the dermis.

Epidermis

The epidermis or top layer is made up of cells that are constantly renewing and shedding, the life cycle of a cell being approximately 30 days. The surface of the skin has a unique ridge pattern that does not change; this is particularly noticable on the finger pads. These ridges help with grip and friction and because of their uniqueness are sometimes used for identicication purposes such as fingerprint matching.

The epidermis has no blood vessels and is formed by five layers or strata of tissue lying on a base membrane. The thickness of the epidermis depends on where it is located on the body. For example, it is thicker on the soles of the feet than around the eye area. It contains pores which are passageways for hair and secretory glands, such as sweat and sebum, and it contains melanocytes that form the pigment melanin, giving the skin its colouring.

The epidermis at the tips of the fingers and toes are formed into nail beds, the living part of nails that are simply hard, keratinized extensions of the epidermis.

Dermis

The dermis or middle layer (thickest part) is the true skin, being connective tissue containing collagen and elastin fibres for strength and elasticity. These fibres are established in an important pattern known as 'Langers lines of cleavage'. If injury is sustained at right angles to the lines, healing will be more difficult and tend to gape, whereas those parallel will mesh together easily. Surgeons will always try to make incisions parallel to these lines to promote healing and reduce scarring.

The dermis layer contains blood, lymph and nerve vessels and the appendages of sweat and sebaceous glands and hair follicles. It is the sensory receptors in the nerve endings that are stimulated during massage treatments. Unlike the epidermis, the dermis does not constantly renew or shed; it does, however, have a repair mechanism when damaged. Fibroblasts found in the layer reproduce and form a patch of new connective tissue commonly known as a scar.

CASE STUDY **SKIN**

CLIENT PROFILE
Shelley is an 18-year-old who suffers with acne. A friend is studying to be a therapist and needs volunteers for practice sessions. As a student, she is wary of Shelley's skin condition but with advice from her tutor and knowledge about the condition, she is happy to include Shelley as one of her subjects.

REGULARITY
Shelley received a massage each week over a period of two months as part of her friend's training programme.

TYPE OF TREATMENT
Many skin lesions may look untreatable but some types, such as severe acne, are not infectious and although the area is contraindicated whilst visibly inflamed or infected, this condition common in puberty and adolescence can be helped by general body massage. This will improve the texture and tone of the skin through promotion of circulation and added nutrients.

OUTCOME
Week by week, Shelley's skin condition showed signs of improvement. The accumulation of dead bacteria and dried sebum slowly reduced and the itching that she sometimes experienced became less frequent.

Layers of the skin The skin is a complex organ composed of two levels: the epidermis and the dermis. The hypodermis is not part of the skin, but connects the skin to the muscle and bone underneath and provides it with nerves and blood vessels.

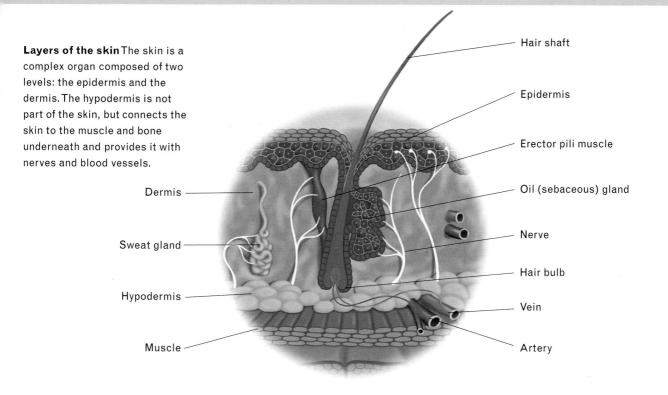

Hair shaft

Epidermis

Erector pili muscle

Oil (sebaceous) gland

Dermis

Nerve

Sweat gland

Hair bulb

Hypodermis

Vein

Muscle

Artery

The dermis also contains bulbs or follicles that contain living hair roots, the shaft or dead part of the hair fibre appearing above the skin. The shape of the follicle in the dermis will mould the shape of the hair as it grows – a straight follicle will produce straight hair, oval will produce wavy hair.

Subcutaneous layer

The subcutaneous layer or hypodermis is not strictly skin but superficial fascia, rich in fat and nerve receptors. The thickness of this fatty layer depends on age and gender; it acts as a cushion against injury and a store for energy.

Functions of the skin

There are many functions but the main ones can be classified in six 'tions': absorption, sensation, protection, immunization, regulation and excretion – ASPIRE ations!

- Absorption is limited because of the skin's natural tendency to repel moisture. However, through a synthesis process, melanocyte cells in the skin convert UV rays in sunlight absorbed through the skin into valuable vitamin D.
- Sensation is an extension of the nervous system that informs the body about external changes such as pain, temperature and pressure. Thousands of nerve endings in the skin send back messages to the brain in order for the body to respond to these changes.

- Protection is one of the main functions of the skin, acting as a barrier against physical injury and biological invasions such as bacteria and viruses.
- Immunization is linked to special cells in the dermis called Langerhans cells. They attach themselves to and destroy pathogens and also trigger immunological reactions with the help of T cells.
- Regulation of the body's temperature to an average 37°C (98.6°F) ensures that the cells function well and homeostasis is maintained, essential to survival. The skin plays a major part in this by adjusting to compensate for any changes. For example, if body temperature rises, the blood vessels in the dermis expand, or dilate, allowing more blood to the travel to the surface of the skin in order to expel body heat. If the body temperature drops, the opposite happens, reducing the amount of heat leaving the body.
- Excretion through the skin occurs when metabolic waste is eliminated through perspiration. Small amounts of body salts are expelled from the body in sweat produced to cool the body down as part of the heat regulation process. The sweat evaporates quickly and acts as a cooling agent. Another excretion is a natural oil produced by the sebaceous glands lining the skins hair follicles called sebum. This oil helps to lubricate and moisturize the skin and hair and prevents them drying out.

Effects of massage on the skin

As a response to massage the small blood vessels in the dermis dilate, producing heat and red pigmentation, which is why a therapist can actually see the effect of their work – the skin being the one organ and system that is actually handled during a treatment. Massage promotes blood supply and nourishes and tones the skin. Certain strokes, in particular friction, stimulate the production of oil or sebum from the sebaceous glands, adding natural oils to the skin, and at the same time increasing activity as an excretory organ for water and waste products. As the nerve endings in the skin are soothed, signals will be sent to the brain to promote relaxation of the whole body.

Perhaps one of the most important affects of massage is to encourage healing where injury has occurred. By helping to realign the collagen in the fibrous tissue, any scar tissue will be strengthened and formed without complications. It can even help with pathological skin conditions where massage is not contraindicated.

Massage for common conditions of the skin

The list here is comprehensive because massage entails constant contact with clients' skin and it is important for you to be able to recognize skin conditions and diseases for the safety of both you and your clients.

Massage is usually contraindicated around the area affected by a skin condition; in viral conditions massage is usually totally contraindicated due to the risk of infection.

Congenital conditions

These are skin conditions that appear from birth, vary in severity and are not contagious.

Eczema

Characterized by redness, water discharge, crusting, itchiness and burning, this inflammatory disorder is not contagious.
Massage: Local contraindication.

Psoriasis

This chronic form of dermatitis is characterized by red, flaky skin covered by thick dry silvery scales. It is found on elbows, knees, backs, scalp and buttocks, and is not contagious.
Massage: Local contraindication.

Pigmentation

Includes age spots, birthmarks, strawberry and port wine marks.
Massage: Not contraindicated.

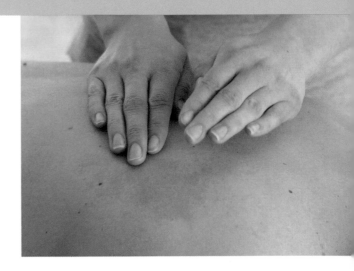

Skin conditions Recognizing skin conditions and their contraindications is of utmost importance when applying safe massage therapy, due to the constant contact with the skin.

Bacterial conditions

Very minute organisms, which are usually not contagious, infect the skins and cause a bacterial infection.

Acne vulgaris and rosacea

Vulgaris is characterized by whiteheads, blackheads, pustules and other debris around the face, back chest and shoulders. A bacterial infection of the hair follicles, it is not contagious. Rosacea is a chronic inflammatory disorder characterized by persistent redness and swelling that affects the face, nose and cheeks. It is not contagious.
Massage: Local contraindication.

Boils

These are characterized by pain, redness and swelling due to an infection that causes inflammation around a hair follicle. They are not contagious.
Massage: Local contraindication.

Folliculitis

A bacterial infection characterized by inflammation of a hair follicle, often in conjunction with acne vulgaris. It is not contagious.
Massage: Local contraindication.

Impetigo

This is characterized by blisters that weep and develop thick yellow crusts around the mouth, nose and hands, mostly in children. It is a highly contagious bacterial infection that can be spread by hand contact and handling contaminated items.
Massage: Contraindicated.

Viral conditions

Poisonous matter attacks the skin and causes a viral condition which is usually highly contagious.

Herpes simplex and zoster

Herpes simplex, also known as a cold sore, is characterized by small blisters around the mouth. It can spread to other parts of the body. It is a viral condition that is very contagious. Herpes zoster, also known as shingles, is the adult form of chickenpox. Characterized by a rash of blisters that cause severe itching and pain, it is a viral condition.
Massage: Contraindicated.

Warts and verrucas

Characterized by a thickening of the epidermis resulting in a growth on the skin, warts are caused by a virus and are highly contagious. A verruca is a form of wart on the foot.
Massage: Local contraindication.

Fungal

A fungus grows or springs up suddenly, it is a spongy outgrowth that is usually highly contagious.

Athlete's foot – tinea pedis

Characterized by discolouration of the skin, red tisssue ridges and skin that may break or discharge with an unpleasant odour, this condition is highly infectious.
Massage: Local contraindication.

Ringworm – tinea corporis

Characterized by a raised red ringed patch that scales and itches, this group of fungal diseases is highly infectious.
Massage: Contraindicated.

Other

These are conditions that do not fit into categories but vary from life-threatening to simple discolourations.

Skin cancer

The most serious type of skin cancer, malignant melanoma, is characterized by the appearance of large, irregular shaped moles, often more than one colour. They sometimes bleed or itch. If you notice a mole larger than 6mm (¼ inch) in diameter you should advise your client to have it checked by their GP.
Massage: With medical consent.

Allergic reactions/dermatitis/hives

When skin is irritated it produces a substance called histamine in defence, which in turn can cause watery eyes, itching, swelling and red blotchy patches. Hives is a severe reaction characterized by the presence of pink wheals. It is important to check at consultation stage that a client has no allergies that may be aggravated by massage or the medium used to apply it.
Massage: Local contraindication.

Bruise

Characterized by swelling and discolouration as a result of ruptured blood vessels under the skin, a bruise is an injury that does not break the skin.
Massage: Local contrainidication.

Ulcers

Skin ulcers or bed sores may occur in bedridden patients or wheelchair users as a result of the constant pressure on small areas of the skin.
Massage: Local contraindication.

Cysts

These are benign swellings under the skin filled with sebum and debris. They frequently become infected and treatment is by surgical incision.
Massage: Local contraindication.

Lice

Head lice are parasitic insects found in the hair and diagnosed by the presence of egg sacs. They are highly contagious.
Massage: Contraindicated.

Scars

These are the result of a natural healing process. They are pink in colour due to the presence of blood vessels.
Massage: Local contraindication until healing process has taken place.

Corns/calluses

These are thickened cone-shaped bumps on the skin, usually found over toe joints as a result of repeated friction or pressure..
Massage: Local contraindication.

Scabies

This is an infestation of parasites under the skin that causes intense itching. It is highly contagious.
Massage: Contraindicated.

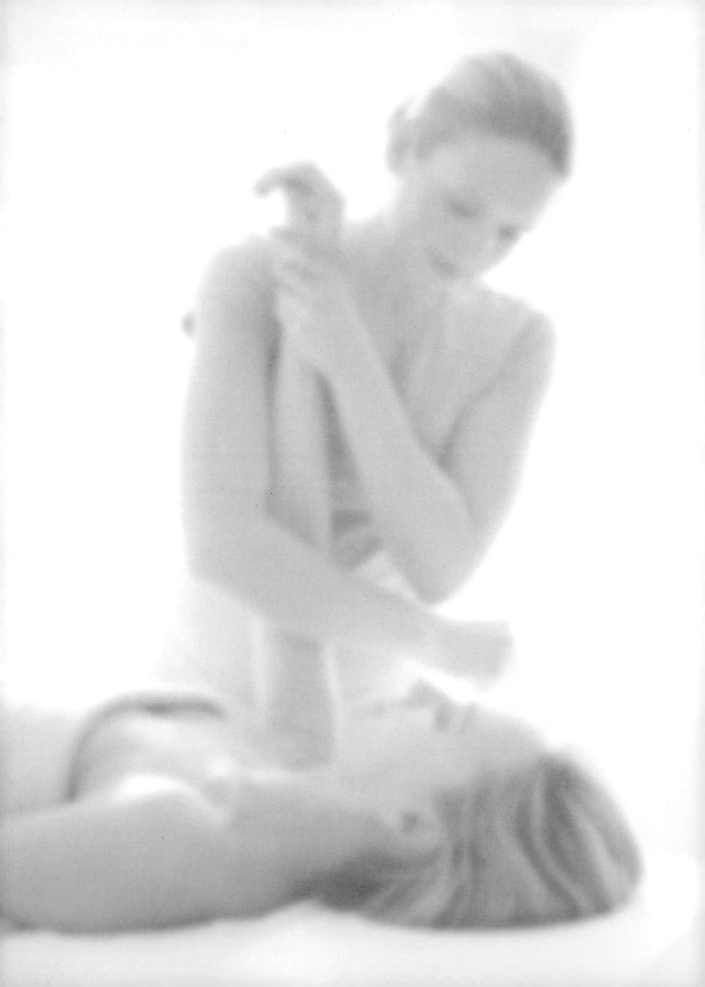

Massage preparation

Thorough preparation prior to massage is essential to make sure that you are ready, the environment is ready and your client is ready. Massage is a two-way interaction and should only be given if both parties are comfortable. Do not try to massage if you are feeling stressed, if your mind is elsewhere, or if you are not in full health. Make sure that everything you need is to hand and that the room is clean and warm. The environs should encourage the client to feel safe, comfortable and relaxed.

Creating the right environment

Preparing the surroundings is an important element in creating the atmosphere of comfort and relaxation central to massage therapy.

The room you use should reflect the image you wish to promote. If you want to specialize in sports and remedial work, for example, your room should have a clinical appearance with clean lines, simple white linens and muscle and skeletal charts for reference. In contrast, a therapist working on general well-being will want to create a warm and relaxing environment with the use of subdued lighting, subtle colour and, perhaps, background music and some homely touches. Many therapists will have a cross-section of clients, so a room that incorporates a little of both will work best.

All rooms should have the basic furnishings of a mirror, clock, supply shelves or cabinet, a wastebin with a lid for hygiene purposes, chairs and stools for client and therapist and a place for the client to store personal items. Windows should have suitable covering to ensure privacy and diffuse light.

Heating

The most important aspect of the environment to get right is the heating. A person's body temperature drops while receiving massage and muscles will not relax in a chilly atmosphere so the room needs to be warmed beforehand. Some fresh air is good but there should not be any draughts.

TAKING CARE OF THE SENSES

Make sure that the massage room has a clean, fresh atmosphere by airing it before treatments. Flowers or essential oil burners can be placed in the room for their aromas, but do make sure that your clients will not react to these. Candles are not recommended in a professional massage room due to the risk of fire and spillage of hot wax.

Aim to maintain the temperature at approximately 24°C (75°F) but keep an electric fan available for those clients who are naturally warm, pregnant or suffer hot flushes, who may find the room too hot. Do not make the mistake of setting the room temperature at a level you, the therapist, feel comfortable working in as the physical exertion involved in massage will push up your body temperature. To keep cool wear loose clothing made of natural fibres that allow the air to circulate and evaporate any perspiration.

Warm the towels before use by placing them on a radiator or in a warmer, and take the chill off your chosen massage medium by placing it in hot water or on a warm surface. If your hands are cold, hold them under running hot water for a short time until they reach a temperature that is comfortable for your client.

Providing a peaceful atmosphere

Some people enjoy background music playing, which helps relaxation into the rhythm of the massage. There are many excellent cds and cassettes widely available specifically for this purpose or the client may wish to provide their own.

Avoid using harsh lighting as this can feel intrusive and the eyes need to relax as well as the rest of the body. Subdued lights such as table lamps are ideal and natural light will probably be enough for morning and daytime treatments. There must be enough light to enable the client to fill out paperwork, undress and dress, safely move around the room and get on and off the massage table. Reasonable light is also needed during the treatment so that the therapist can assess skin condition.

Before you start

Before each session check you have everything to hand so you will not need to break your concentration. Besides your table and related accessories you will need massage media, linens, couch roll, pillow and bolsters, as well as a thin blanket or throw if it is winter. Do not forget to provide drinking water for after the massage and a box of tissues or kitchen roll may also come in handy.

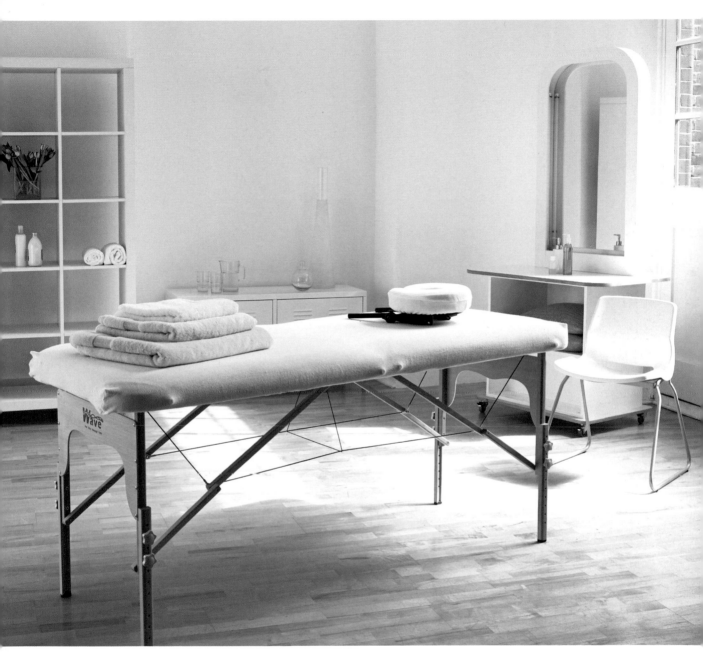

Other thoughtful items are some basic cosmetic supplies for client use such as contact-lens solution, make-up remover and pads. You will also need cleaning supplies, waterless anti-bacterial handwash, ice packs and basic first-aid items including some mints or candy in the case of a diabetic emergency.

Make sure you are comfortable in the footwear and clothes you are wearing. Sleeves should be short or rolled up out of the way and any jewellery, rings or watch removed. You cannot massage with long nails and rough skin will feel very abrasive to the client so make sure your

Professional environment A treatment room should promote relaxation but at the same time be clinical with clean lines. Subdued lighting and colours will create a warm and inviting environment for any type of massage treatment.

hands are well manicured and moisturized. Tie back any long hair and do not forget that you will be working very close to your client – if you have indulged in food and drink that might have unpleasant after-effects on your breath use mouthwash or breath fresheners.

Equipment

Hands are not the only tools of the trade for the massage therapist. The skills learnt are enhanced by using the correct equipment in a professional manner. This includes a massage table or chair and related accessories that should be regularly maintained.

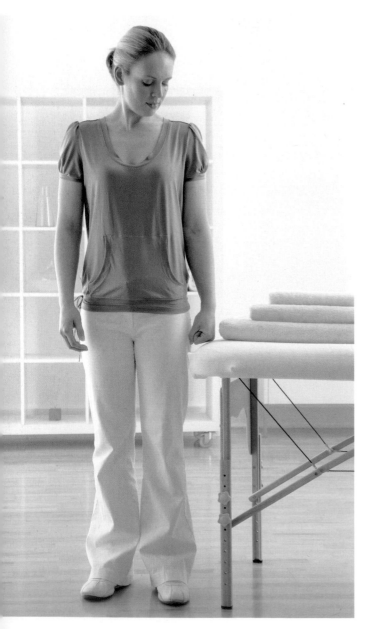

The massage table

The largest and most expensive piece of equipment you will ever have to purchase or replace is your massage table. There is an enormously wide range of professional massage tables available, with a variety of colours, padding, fabric, weights and even shapes.

Most are lightweight, portable and easy to store, but if you have the luxury of your own permanent massage space one of the sturdy stationary tables is the better option. For comfort and safety and to feel confident in your table, purchase the best you can afford from a reputable table manufacturer who will give you a warranty and aftercare service.

When choosing your table, the first dimension to check is the width. Tables range from 70–80 cm (28–32 inches) wide, but what you have to remember is that this is the width of the frame; the padding and covering can add a further 2–8 cm (1–3 inches) to this measurement. A table less than 70 cm (28 inches) wide will make clients feel uneasy and they may not be able to rest their arms comfortably on side of their torso. It would also not be a suitable table for treating pregnant clients.

At the other end of the scale, wider than 80 cm (32 inches) would make it difficult for you to work the opposite side of the client and apply pressure without overstretching, unless you are very long bodied. Taking into account your own height, range of movement and the ease of picking up and transporting the table, choose a width within the normal range and try before you buy.

Next look at the height of the table. Cheaper models generally have a fixed height but, it is advisable always to buy a table where the height can be adjusted to suit by lengthening or shortening the four legs. To find out your

Massage table Once you have chosen your table it will need adjusting to the correct working height to enable easy range of movement and pressure without overstretching.

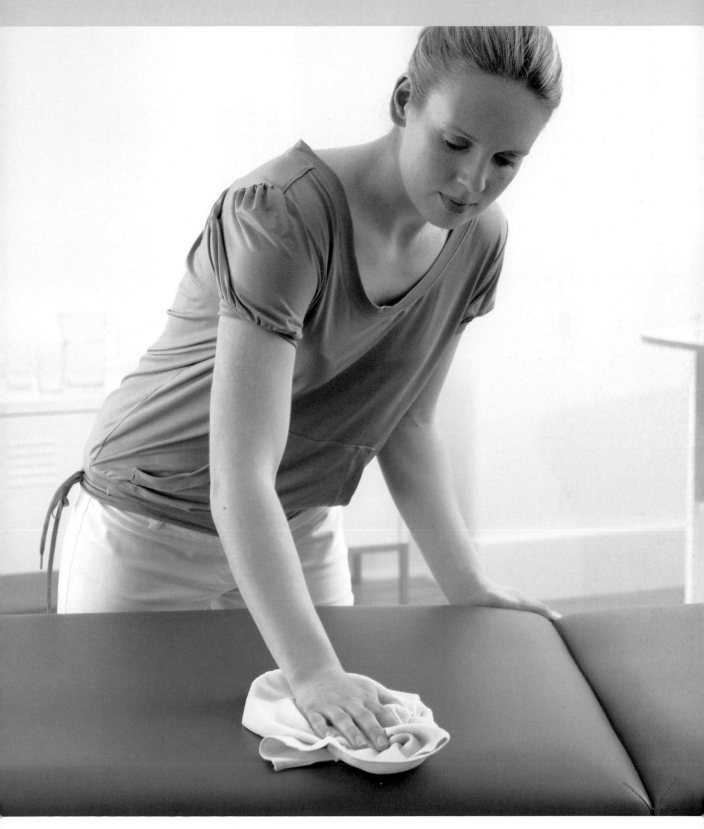

Keeping clean The most expensive piece of equipment you
will buy is a massage table and a daily clean with a soft, dry
cloth should keep it in good condition.

correct working height, stand upright next to a table in the footwear you generally wear when massaging and drop your arms by your side. Where your knuckles brush the top of the table is your optimal height.

As you become more experienced, you may wish to vary the height slightly, enabling you to lean into the muscle more and apply deeper pressure. For therapists practising deep-tissue massage, the correct table height is where the tips of the fingertips on an extended hand brush the surface instead of the knuckles. When practising other therapies such as craniosacral therapy and reiki you may require the flexibility of working at a higher height than for massage.

Massage tables are a standard length of 183–185 cm (72–73 inches), which will fit most clients. A face cradle will add a further 25–30 cm (10–12 inches) to the length while the client is in a prone position and if you regularly treat very tall clients, most models of tables sell extensions that can be easily attached and detached to the end of the table.

Table frames are generally made either from wood or aluminium, the latter being the lightest and usually quicker to adjust in height.

The main points to check if you are able visit a showroom or exhibition to select your purchase are the padding and stability, as these are the two things that clients will remember after their visit. The denser and thicker the padding on top of your massage table frame, the more comfortable it will feel to your client. Table pads in general last an average of five years before starting to lose resilience, and multi-layered designs will last longer than single-layered ones.

After regular use some models of table loosen at the joints and may wobble or creak as you apply pressure stokes. This can be disconcerting and annoying to the client, so check the lateral stability of the showroom model by grabbing one end of the table and rocking it back and forth. Most models have stability wires that can be tightened on a regular basis and wood-framed tables can be oiled around the joints to prevent noise and excess movement.

All tables come covered with a specialized vinyl that does not perish if covered in oil, however it can be ripped by sharp implements and so care is needed when cleaning or handling. There is also a luxury vinyl substitute available that is strong and durable but more expensive. Do not be seduced by a particular colour of table; the majority of the time it will be covered with a couch cover and towels or is tucked away in a carry bag.

Once you have made your purchase, keep it in good condition with regular care. The vinyl should only come into contact with oil or body fluids if no protective drape has been used or there is seepage. A daily wipe down after the last treatment with a dry, soft non-abrasive cloth should keep it in condition. However if you do need to clean deeper, use a gentle product that is alcohol and bleach free and only clean with disinfectant if there are unidentifiable substances present.

Accessories

A *face cradle* is the horseshoe cushion and frame that attaches at the head of the table, 'cradling' the client's face while in prone position. A standard cradle has one position, parallel to the top of the table, whereas more deluxe models can be adjusted to the comfort of the

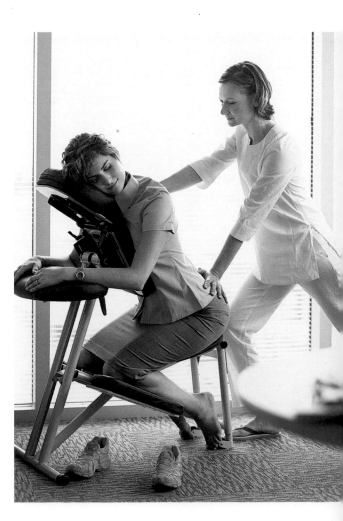

Seated massage Massage chairs were specifically designed over 20 years ago for the application of seated massage, allowing the therapist to offer a very dynamic treatment.

Face cradle A face cradle is used to support the client's head whilst in the prone position, allowing the therapist greater access to the neck and shoulder areas.

client. A face cradle will allow you easier access around the neck and shoulder areas than a face hole built into the table top. Clients are also not always comfortable using a built-in face hole.

Width and length extensions need only be purchased if you have regular clients that require a wider or longer table. Before investing in these accessories make sure that your massage room accommodates the extended size of table and that you still have enough room to manoeuvre easily around the table.

Carrying cases often come as part of the sale package. If you cannot leave your table in situ, the case protects the fabric from damage and temperature changes and also has storage pockets for your massage oils, couch roll and other tools of the trade. Many therapists are mobile and need a case to make the table easier to lift and carry when transporting it between clients.

Bolsters and pillows

Bolsters offer the client support under the knees or ankles when required. The general rule is to support the ankles while lying face down and the knees when face up. A small pillow is also useful to support the neck in supine position. Bolsters and pillows come in a variety of shapes, sizes and fillings to suit individual needs but useful bolster sizes are 66 cm long (26 inches) by 8, 15 or 20 cm (3, 6 or 8 inches) wide. Flat-bottomed bolsters remain in position better than totally round ones. If you cannot afford a bolster initially, a rolled up towel will offer support.

It is a good idea to always keep three or four regular bed pillows available to support clients while they are lying on their side if they are unable to lie in classical positions.

Working without a table

If you are working on the floor, the ideal surface is a futon – a Japanese mattress or massage mat – but a thick duvet or blankets make excellent substitutes. Make sure that whatever you use has enough space for the client and more to save your knees when moving around. Never massage on a bed as it does not have the necessary support required for the client and makes it impossible for you to move easily around the body.

If working on a chair make sure that it is sturdy and that you have a couple of pillows for comfort and support.

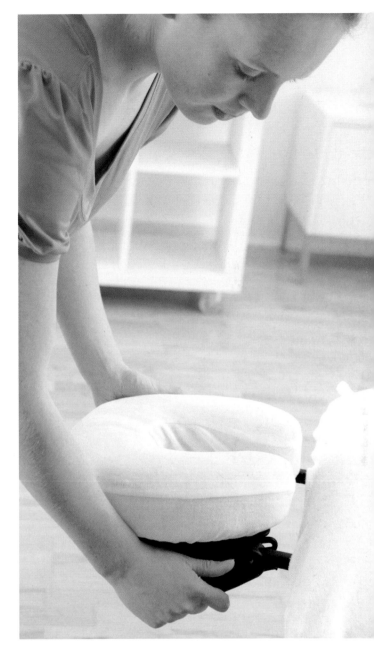

You can buy professional portable massage chairs, designed in the 1980s specifically for seated massage. These have grown in popularity and can be particularly useful when massage is offered in corporate or commercial settings and applied through the clothes. If purchasing a chair it is important that it is light to carry, but sturdy and simple to set up and take down. The adjusters, of which there are several, should be easy to use and robust. The use of face covers will protect the headrest and aftercare is the same as that for a table.

Massage media

Most massage treatments require a lubricant to allow the hands to work smoothly and evenly over the skin. This is usually in the form of an oil, although lotions, creams, waxes and sometimes powders are also used. All these are known as massage media.

How much massage medium to use will depend on the size of your client, how hairy they are, and the dryness of the skin, but in general approximately 50 ml or 50 g (3 tablespoons/2 oz) is needed for a whole body massage. It may take a little practice to get it right; most students tend to use too much at first, which makes it difficult to get good contact. The aim is to use just a thin film which will be absorbed after the treatment.

When buying a massage oil, sometimes known as a base or carrier oil, choose the best quality that you can afford. There are many different types available at varying prices depending on their source and each have their own unique properties. Sunflower, grapeseed, sweet almond and jojoba are commonly used. There is no need to worry about nut allergies as you are only applying oil externally and the penetration is superficial, but if in doubt do a patch test on a new client by rubbing a drop of oil on the inner elbow or wrist a day or two before their appointment and check for any reaction. Some baby oils that include lanolin or mineral oil may cause a skin reaction and tend to absorb less easily. These oils are not suitable for professional massage purposes as they clog the pores and deplete the skin's natural nutrients.

Prepare the oil beforehand by decanting it into a suitable vessel. The easiest and least messy method of dispensing oil is to keep it in a small plastic bottle with a flip top. An alternative is to pour some into a wide rimmed bowl that you can dip your fingers into.

Other media, such as a massage lotions, creams or waxes, can be pleasant to use, particularly on dry skin or areas such as the feet, but highly perfumed cosmetic body lotions should be avoided – they are not suitable for massage. Talcum powder is particularly useful when applying strokes that do not require much glide.

Aromatherapy oils

You may be tempted to buy aromatherapy or essential oils to add a further dimension to your massage; however, there are some cautions. These oils are very concentrated and powerful, and many have contraindications. A therapist should consult a qualified aromatherapist if they want to introduce essential oils to a treatment. Never apply them neat to the skin and always mix with a carrier oil in a ratio of 1 to 20. For example, in 10ml of base oil use a maximum of five drops of essential oil.

There are many good quality, pre-blended oils readily available and this is the safest and most economical way to enhance a massage treatment. If you want to mix your own make sure you only prepare enough for a single treatment, as oils exposed to the atmosphere oxidize rapidly and become rancid. Aromatherapy oils are sensitive to light and should be stored in dark bottles so as not to destroy their properties.

Application

Remember to warm the massage medium and your hands before making contact with the skin. If using oil, place the container in hot water for a few minutes or close to a heater. Position the dispenser close to the massage table for easy access, but do not be tempted to place it on the client's drapes.

There are various ways to apply oil, the most common being to pour a small amount, roughly half a teaspoon, into the palm of one hand and then rub the palms together to spread the oil evenly. Do this with your hands slightly away from the client.

The best way to apply more oil during the treatment without disrupting the flow is to leave one hand on the body and slowly pour the oil over the back of the hand, then glide the flat of your other hand across, spreading it on the body. Alternatively, turn your contact hand upwards and slightly cupped, then pour the required oil into the palm. This has the added benefit of re-oiling both hands when gliding the other hand over.

The confidence with which you contact and apply oil during the treatment is very important. The aim is for that first touch to feel relaxed and reassuring, transmitting the message that this is the start of the treatment and enabling the client to adjust to your touch. Never break contact with your client during a massage – always have

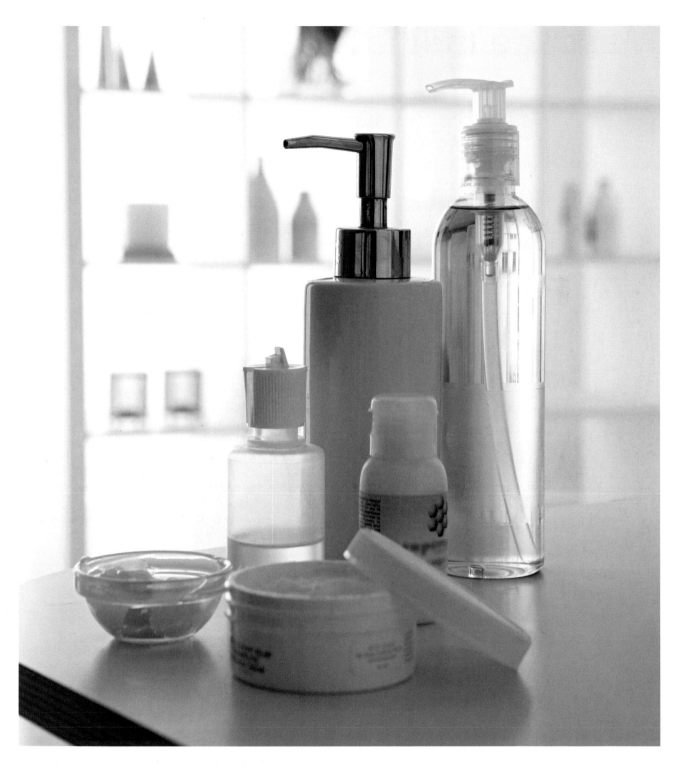

one hand placed on them throughout. If, for some reason, you need to break and re-establish contact, make sure this is carried out in a gentle and smooth manner, keeping the flow of the massage and not leaving the client wondering whether the massage has finished or not.

Massage media There is a wide choice of massage media, including oils, creams, lotions, powder and natural waxes. Each therapist and client will have their personal preferences.

Professionalism

The image that you convey to clients and the way you conduct your business ethically will demonstrate your professionalism. Your technical ability is reflected in your attitude, communication, confidentiality and your ability to work within a code of conduct. Any crossing of these boundaries would be considered unprofessional.

The results of our actions can have major impact on clients and so it is important to remain professional at all times. Bear in mind that you can also be unprofessional without being unethical. The therapist that chews gum in front of a client, for example, is not violating any ethical code but it would be considered unprofessional behaviour.

The initial consultation with a client sets a professional tone from the start, and, along with communication, this will form the basis of your therapeutic relationship. Remember that you are creating a reputable image not only for your practice but for the profession as a whole; an uncaring first massage may leave a poor image of massage in general with a new client and there may not be a second chance to remedy this.

Dress is important; wearing clothing that separates you as the therapist and projects a clinical image will help instil confidence and trust, particularly in clients of the opposite sex. Medical scrubs and coats or smart sportswear are ideal as they allow for freedom of movement without being overflowing and are easy to launder. Keep to simple colours and change daily. Hair should be clean and tied back, facial hair neat and well groomed, fingernails clean and short and because of the closeness of contact, attention to personal hygiene and fresh breath is imperative.

A code of ethics lays down conduct guidelines that a therapist works within. They may be personal guidelines formulated by yourself but more often they are set by professional organizations or training establishments, and play a major part in the regulatory process. These educate us in the consequences when having to make professional decisions. Common principles laid down in such codes include guidelines on:

- **Confidentiality** – the safekeeping of privileged information and the client's right to and guarantee of privacy. It is both unethical and illegal to breach this trust.
- **Discrimination** – covering areas of gender, age, race, religion and sexual practices, this also comes within the realms of statutory law.
- **Informed consent** – giving the client enough knowledge for them to agree to your services and make an informed decision on treatment.
- **Best practice** – making available the highest quality of care and safety to each client, staying within the limits of your training and qualifications.
- **Professional boundaries** – avoiding any conflict of interest and if necessary referring the client to another therapist where dual relationships occur.
- **Contact issues** – avoiding initiating any contact or communication that could be considered to be of a sexual nature. Poor draping methods, massaging or touching intimate areas and wearing unsuitable clothing are considered unethical; sexually related comments are totally prohibited.
- **Laws and legislation** – you are expected not only to follow the rules set out by your member organization, but also to work within statutory law. It is also your duty to report any known professional misconduct to the appropriate authorities.
- **Continual professional development (CPD)** – It is a requirement to continue your massage education after qualification so that you remain informed of new trends and techniques and develop underpinning knowledge that will benefit your clients.

Being a member of an association or body and following their set Code of Ethics may not be statutory but has many benefits and protects you and your clients. During your career you may have to make decisions on ethical grounds and question the outcome of that decision. In a situation where there is vagueness and it is difficult to

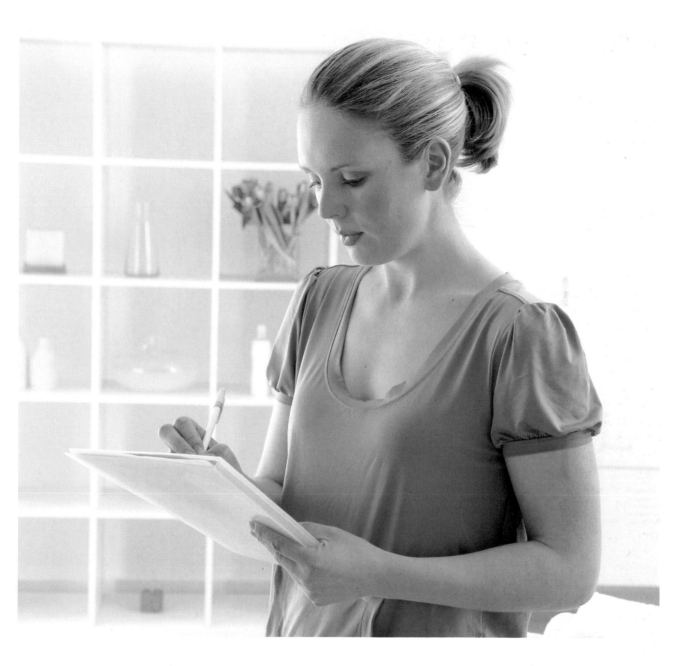

decide which action will do the least harm and the most good, the ethics committee of your chosen association will be able to advise and support you on the decision you make.

Boundaries

Your professionalism also depends on an awareness of your boundaries and limitations and being sensitive to those of your clients. Inevitably you will learn this through experience rather than from a textbook, but issues you should consider include:

Professional image Your image is one of the first things a new client will register on meeting you, so this plays a major part in setting a professional tone.

- handling appointments and 'no shows'
- preparation and setting for the treatment
- dealing with unsatisfied clients
- physical contact and personal space between you and the client

- keeping a professional distance
- integrity and maintaining moral and artistic values
- learning to say no to treating a client
- terminating a session in extreme circumstances
- client neglect or abuse whether unintentional or deliberate.

Examples of common mistakes involving the crossing of professional boundaries are as follows:

- Working outside the limits of your professional training: After taking a weekend workshop, a therapist is eager to incorporate new techniques into treatments immediately without having the practice and hands-on experience required to carry them out safely. This could result in injury to a client and would be considered client neglect. Perfect the skills before integrating them into a professional, remunerated treatment.
- Responding to emotional release: A massage therapist is not trained in psychology and can give a sympathetic ear but not advice. Offer referral details to a qualified counsellor but only on the request of the client.
- Making personal comments: You should refrain from making any comments about a client's personal appearance; a careless phrase or gesture, however complimentary, can be misread.
- Having dual relationships: A client who is a friend, or a client who becomes a friend, makes the therapeutic relationship vulnerable. Both parties are open to the dangers of neglect and the transference and countertransference of feelings, unresolved issues, personal needs and emotions. The decision to start a romantic or physical relationship with an ex-client should be considered very carefully as it can damage the reputation of the therapist and may unnerve existing clients. Best practice is not to start a relationship of this nature, but if it is unavoidable, a period of six months between the therapist terminating the therapeutic relationship and starting the personal one is recommended.

The cornerstone of professionalism is self-accountability. Be honest with yourself about who you are and what you do out of sight of others. As you develop your self-accountability skills you will be able to consider and accept the consequences of your actions. The ethics you apply to your personal life are the bench marks and warning bells in your professional role. For example, if you find it difficult to keep secrets in general,

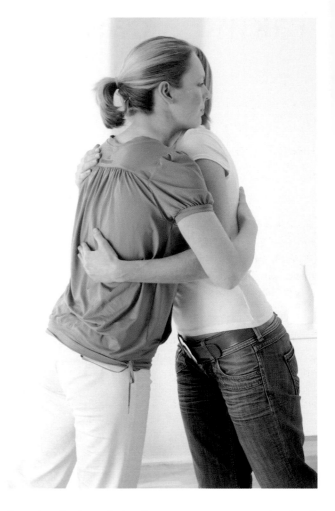

Crossing the boundaries Be aware not to cross professional boundaries. This type of greeting or farewell is not appropriate between a massage therapist and client.

you will have to watch yourself carefully in client confidentiality matters.

The use of a mentor or clinical supervisor protects both the therapist and client by providing an ethical arena in which matters relating to therapeutic relationships can be discussed and to offer support and guidance. This is the correct place for a therapist to be nurtured and receive appreciation for their work. It is a valuable education tool and practised widely by body workers, physical therapists and other somatic practitioners.

Many therapists fall into the trap of being genuinely concerned for their clients but neglect to develop their professional image. A good therapist will combine their outward professionalism and their internal integrity to the benefit of their clients.

Taking a case history

An essential part of a first appointment is the gathering of information on your client's medical history and lifestyle, assessment and planning. The expectations of the client also need to be established; therapists that develop a large clientele often use the knowledge gleaned to exceed that expectation.

The primary purpose of taking a case history is to construct a holistic picture of your client's health, highlighting problem areas on which to base a safe treatment plan. The consultation itself should take no longer than 15 minutes on the first visit and the client should be made aware on booking that this will take place and adjust the time of their appointment accordingly.

On subsequent appointments a simple update of any changes or incidences since the last massage need only take five minutes. You may wish to create your own case-history forms as the basis of your client record, although there are pre-printed sheets available through massage supply stores. If the client is able to claim any part of the treatment as part of a medical insurance, the third-party payers will have their own forms for you to use.

The case-history sheet should be easy to read, organized logically, contain only relevant questions and made easy to complete. Questions should include contact details, date of birth, physician contacts and an emergency number. It is useful to know if the client has had any previous massage experience and some lifestyle information, but this is not imperative. It is very important to know whether they are on medication and under medical supervision, and whether they have any historical or present medical conditions that may contraindicate massage. An example sheet is shown on page 100. To speed up the process, ask the client to fill in the contact details section as they arrive for their appointment.

It is important to establish a professional relationship at this stage as it is your first contact. The environment you choose for the consultation process needs to put the client at ease so that they are happy to impart the information you require. A prominent display of qualification and insurance certificates will indicate that you are serious about your role as a therapist and send out positive signals. The massage treatment room is ideal for this purpose but if it is not available, find a quiet area where you can discuss details in private and uninterrupted. If using the treatment room, make sure there are comfortable chairs available and it goes without saying, the client should remain fully clothed for the consultation.

To get the most from a consultation, start with the more general questions, moving on to the more complicated medical ones. By filling in the case-history sheet yourself, extra questions can be asked where more information or clarification is required. You can also ask the client to confirm why they have come for a massage and the type of treatment they would like. Be aware that a client may not wish to spend more than ten minutes on this, so speed is of the essence and some clients may be unwilling to give any information. In this case, note down any relevant answers they may have given in conversation and make a decision to treat or not.

Be confident and professional in your delivery, reassuring the client that all information remains totally confidential, is stored safely and used only to plan a safe and beneficial treatment unique to them.

Records should be updated after each visit, documenting time and dates, the treatment given and any observations. Your insurance company may need to have sight of this information in the event of a dispute. Keeping records is discussed in more detail on page 240.

The final part of the consultation is to explain what the treatment will involve. Reassure your client that their modesty will be preserved with drapes at all times and only the area being worked on will be exposed at any time. Show them where they can store their clothes and belongings and ask them to remove all clothing and jewellery and place themselves on the table in your starting position, covered with a towel. Leave the room while this happens, knocking before re-entering so as not to cause embarrassment. If a client feels more comfortable retaining their underwear, agree to their request and adapt your massage accordingly.

Client form

Name _____ Date of consultation _____

Address _____

Telephone _____

Date of birth _____ Occupation _____

Before the treatment

To avoid a low blood sugar level, please ensure that you have eaten something within the 3 hours preceding treatment, but do not have a large meal, any alcohol or non-prescription medication in the hour preceding treatment.

Please tick any of the following that apply to you and discuss them with your practitioner.

- ☐ under the care of a doctor/other practitioner
- ☐ taking any prescribed medication
- ☐ pregnant or trying to conceive
- ☐ neck injury
- ☐ stiff neck
- ☐ back injury

- ☐ backache or pain (upper/mid/lower back)
- ☐ muscle cramps
- ☐ pulled muscle
- ☐ dislocation
- ☐ fracture
- ☐ other injury
- ☐ recent surgery
- ☐ recent hospitalisation

- ☐ recent scar tissue
- ☐ cuts/bruises
- ☐ skin or scalp condition
- ☐ poor circulation
- ☐ thrombosis
- ☐ varicose veins
- ☐ heart trouble
- ☐ high blood pressure
- ☐ low blood pressure

- ☐ arthritis/rheumatism
- ☐ asthma
- ☐ diabetes
- ☐ epilepsy
- ☐ osteoporosis
- ☐ cancer
- ☐ any contagious or infectious condition
- ☐ any other serious illness

Practitioner notes _____

_____

_____

_____

After the treatment

Everyone has a slightly different experience of this type of massage. Take a few movements to feel the effects and discuss them with your practitioner if you wish. Please remember to drink plenty of water after the treatment.

Please sign and date the following statement

I confirm that I have read the above statement and discussed it with my practitioner. I am aware that it is neither diagnostic nor remedial, nor is it a cure or a substitute for medical treatment. I confirm that I have not omitted any information concerning my health that should properly be disclosed and I accept full responsibility for advising my practitioner of any changes to my medical circumstances which may arise in the future.

Signature of client _____ Date _____

I confirm that your personal details and all information imparted during our consultation will be treated with the utmost confidentiality.

Signature of practitioner _____ Date _____

What do you hope to experience as a result of massage? _____

_____

Practitioner to note Client Preferences _____

_____

Please briefly explain all checked items _____

_____

Assessing the client's needs

Each massage session is unique to the individual client and you will need to prepare a treatment plan or 'map' to make sure the outcome is beneficial. The plan acts as a framework around which the massage is based.

Assessment involves piecing together all the information you have gathered on a client's condition – including their expectations – and planning is the strategy and outline of the steps you will follow throughout the massage. Relying on memory is not enough – a written plan, however brief, is good practice.

An informed assessment covers the purpose of the massage, any pain or discomfort present, allergies or skin conditions, lifestyle and medical history.

When questioning a client about pain or discomfort it is useful to ask them to place it on a scale of 1–10, 1 being the least painful and 10 being the most acute level. You will also need to know when it started, how often it occurs, what aggravates it, the core site and areas it radiates to, what type of pain it is and what, if anything, relieves it.

Information on allergies and skin conditions can be collated from the case history and observations whilst applying massage, but it is important to know before the treatment if they have any allergy to the ingredients of the massage medium you wish to use.

As you collate all this information, you will also be screening the client for any contraindications to massage.

You will need to reassess your finding after each subsequent treatment and document it together with your treatment plan, its execution and the outcome.

The two most popular client note formats used for massage are known as SOAP (Subjective, Objective, Assessment, Plan) notes and APIE (Assessment, Plan, Implementation, Evaluation) notes. You can use either type according to personal preference or in line with other therapists you work with, but in both formats the notes should be short and to the point.

A good treatment plan should include:

- the techniques and areas you are going to use and avoid
- suggested activities and self-care to take up between appointments, such as mineral baths, ice or heat packs, stress reduction – make sure you are not overstepping your professional or statutory limits
- recommended duration and frequency of receiving massage that would be beneficial
- the need for a referral to another trained professional such as an osteopath, physiotherapist or nutritionalist to deal with problems outside your area of expertise.

You may also want to make notes relating to special requirements, for example a client needing assistance, extra support or other complementary therapies. Suggested reading materials may also be appreciated by the client so they become more informed about their conditions.

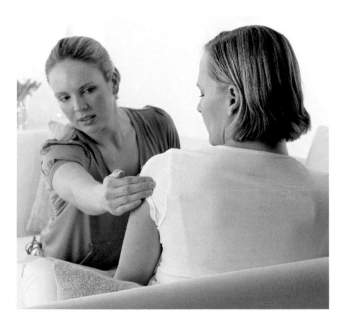

Making an assessment An informed discussion with your client before the massage is essential for finding out information, such as sources of pain or injury.

Importance of communication

Clear communication forms the basis for any successful client–therapist relationship, and is essential in avoiding misunderstandings. Communication skills take time to develop and some people are naturally better at it than others. A newly qualified therapist may benefit from training in communication and awareness skills.

There are a variety of styles that can be used to convey information to a client. The safest method is to employ as many as possible to get your message across. For example, if you are describing a condition you can explain it verbally, use charts and diagrams, give a written handout and invite questions.

Good communication will maintain your working boundaries both verbally and through your body language and behaviour. Boundary issues are always sensitive and subject to misunderstandings. Practical issues, such as making sure your clients understand your normal working hours, may be easy to deal with, whereas issues such as body odour and money can be emotionally challenging and require a clear and sensitive approach.

Power dynamics

A change of power dynamic between the therapist and client can escalate any existing communication problems. Under normal circumstances the therapist is in a superior position to the client; you hold the technical knowhow and knowledge about the treatment. If there is a shift of power, however, because you feel the client has greater knowledge, for example, communication can break down and the outcome of the treatment may be unsatisfactory.

A client may even resent a power dynamic and become reactive, challenging your competence. If you find yourself bowing to a client's demands and becoming resentful (e.g. working outside normal hours or deferring payments), you need to re-evaluate the dynamic and change your style of communication to redress the balance.

Remember to always treat your client as a person not an object, even if it is the end of a very long day. If a client feels that you are listening to them, they will be more open and able to give you the information required to effect a good treatment. Make it comfortable for them to give feedback on any concerns during the treatment and any discomfort they may be feeling.

Body language

Be aware of your client's body language: it can reinforce what is being said or not said. For example, a client may reply that they are comfortable with the pressure of your stroke when asked, but at the same time tense up at your touch. It is important to recognize the conflicting signals and act on them accordingly.

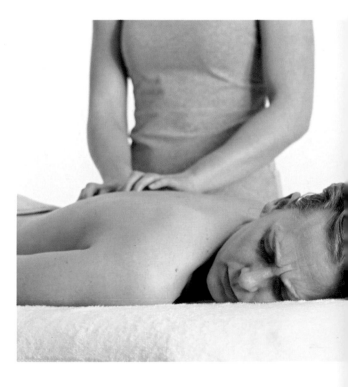

Non-verbal communication Always check that the pressure you are applying is comfortable for the client and adjust it according to the type of stroke and their response.

ARE YOU LISTENING?

The key skill to effective communication is listening. It is not enough just to listen to what the client is saying, you must also understand what it means to the speaker. Search for the core of the message by summarizing it in a word or phrase. For example, if a client says 'Can you do that a little different?' you may hear a request for a different technique, whereas what the message really says is 'I don't like what you are doing, it does not match my expectation.'

Expression of emotion

One of the most important times for effective communication is when emotional expression occurs during a treatment. Hands-on therapies can sometimes provoke strong emotional reflexes that result in crying, anxiety attacks or anger. How you respond and what you say in this situation can make or break the therapeutic relationship. Getting it wrong may even lose you a client in extreme circumstances.

Sometimes touching a specific area can trigger an emotional response associated with a negative past occurrence that you are not aware of. If this happens make sure you keep the client focused on the present. Suggest they open their eyes, take some deep breaths and try to relax. Ask if they would like to terminate the session. If they want you to continue, proceed carefully and refrain from asking any probing questions unrelated to carrying out a safe treatment. Unless you have strong communication skills, defuse the situation by bringing the focus back round to the treatment.

If you find the emotional outbursts overwhelming, you should stop the session and leave the room, putting some distance back in the therapeutic relationship.

Anxiety and fear is sometimes the result of energy moving around the body faster than the person can absorb. The visual signs may be clenching the fists, shallow breathing, trembling, sweating or loss of skin tone. Be aware of these changes and communicate your concerns gently, asking if they are feeling anxious. Slow down the pace of the massage and temporarily

Post-massage communication Make sure you get feedback from your client after massage therapy and practise skillful listening and communication.

pause until the feelings have passed. Focus verbal communication on the actual anxiety, ask where it is felt, whether the sensation is subsiding, etc. If the client is unable to feel more comfortable you should take the decision to stop the treatment.

The most challenging reaction for the massage therapist is that of an angry client. It may take all your communication skills to calm the situation. It is essential that you acknowledge what the client is saying and listen, whether you agree with the reason for the anger or not. Anger provoked by an unconscious memory should be handled carefully, with assistance if necessary. Anger due to poor communication or bad practice should be dealt with calmly and responded to later.

If the client's concerns are valid, an acknowledgement and apology would be appropriate at the next session. If the client was mistaken, however, allow a cooling-off period before explaining that your actions could have been misinterpreted. This will probably be the most delicate situation you have to handle and clear communication is essential.

Skilful listening and communication will enhance the outcome of your massage treatments, maintain ethical practice and keep a healthy connection between you and your clients.

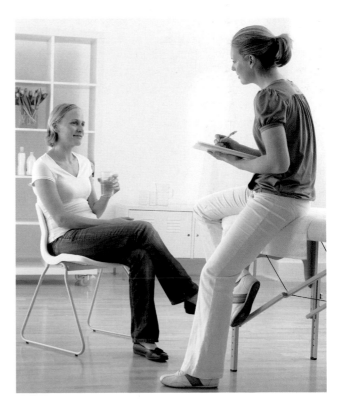

When you should not massage

Massage is one of the safest, least intrusive of complementary therapies. However, there are three categories of basic contraindications that should be borne in mind.

Total contraindication

Massage should not be used for:

- Anyone weak or clinically exhausted, for example, suffering or recovering from a viral infection.
- A person with a high temperature or contagious disease.
- Someone with an infectious skin complaints such as scabies, herpes or warts.
- After surgery, wait 12 months for major and six months for minor operations before treating; scar tissue should be fully healed but if in doubt seek medical practitioner approval.
- Where inflammation is widespread or a condition represents a medical emergency.
- Where a person is under the influence of alcohol or unprescribed drugs.

Localized contraindications

Do not massage:

- The site of a recent fracture, strain or sprain. In these cases work one joint above.

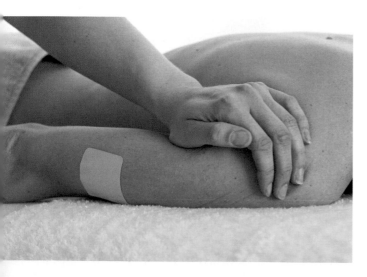

- Areas of surface skin problems such as scar tissue, bruising, tender or inflamed areas and varicose veins. You can work with care above the site and on other unaffected parts of the body.
- In the presence of an abnormal finding, for example, lumps, masses or moles.
- With very deep pressure in pregnancy (after the first trimester), particularly on the lower back and inside leg from ankle to groin.

Medical contraindications

Massage should not be used in:

- Serious medical conditions such as cancer, heart disorders, thrombosis or any condition being treated by a physician that advises against massage.
- The first trimester of pregnancy (see page 184).
- Around areas of injections for at least ten days after the last injection as massage could increase the absorption rate of the medication.

Modifications to your treatments may be necessary if a client is on prescribed medication, including anti-inflammatory drugs, muscle relaxers, narcotic analgesics, corticosteroids, antidepressants, anticoagulants and transdermal patches. Always have a current copy of a prescribing guide (such as MIMMS) to hand to identify types of medication.

It is also not advisable to give massage after a heavy meal. This will make the experience uncomfortable and may have unpleasant after-effects. The general rule is trust your own judgement and common sense. It is a therapist's duty and mark of competency to identify conditions that preclude massage. If a client does not wish to disclose their medical history, the therapist has the right to refuse treatment, the rule being if there is a doubt, do not massage.

Contraindication? If the client is wearing a transdermal patch, always massage above the site of the patch in order to avoid any unnecessary stimulation.

Safety

Although massage is usually a safe therapy, there are a few guidelines to promote the safety of both client and therapist. Apply common-sense procedures and if unsure, do not treat.

As the therapist is generally treating a person who is unclothed there is a risk of transferring pathogens – biological agents capable of causing disease – particularly if working in a hospital environment. Fungi, bacteria and viruses can be transferred by the therapist from one part of a body to another. For example a foot fungus may be transferred to another part of the body by massage.

To avoid this it is advisable to follow certain precautions, such as hand-washing with an antibacterial agent, using gloves where necessary, effective laundering of linens and uniforms, cleaning and disinfecting equipment, ensuring the correct disposal of materials and maintaining the cleanliness of the treatment room.

It is unlikely that there will be contact with body fluids during massage as areas of skin conditions, wounds and lesions are contraindicated. A client or therapist may cough or sneeze or, in extreme conditions, vomit, but employing sanitary procedures should suffice.

Common-sense procedures include: hand wash before and after treatment, wear no jewellery, keep fingernails clean, short and polish free, keep hair clean and tied back, use clean drapes for each treatment, wear a clean uniform every day. Do not be tempted to work if you are feeling ill or suffering from a cold or fever and definitely do not work under the influence of alcohol or other stimulants. Avoid treating clients who are feeling unwell.

Make sure that the toilet facilities are sanitized, have hot and cold water and a good supply of hand-cleaning materials. Finally, ensure that your first aid box is complete and that your first-aid training is up to date.

Vaccinations

In some environments it may be useful for a massage therapist to make sure their immunizations or vaccinations are up to date against tuberculosis and hepatitis B, for example. This may apply more to working in a medical environment than in a private practice.

Use of gloves

The use of disposable gloves is sometimes recommended if the therapist has a cut or open wound, or when handling any contaminated linen and disinfecting massage equipment. And occasionally a client will request that gloves are used. The gloves should be a tight fit to maintain sensitivity, and a water-based lubricant should be used rather than oil-based products, which will break down the latex. You should also be aware that gloves increase friction and may be uncomfortable to the client, particularly if they are hirsute.

If you are not happy to massage in a certain situation unless wearing gloves, you need to discuss the reasons for glove use with the client. This can be a very sensitive situation and you need to make sure that you do not cause offence. Involve the client in the decision and get a firm agreement before the treatment. On no account should you proceed, hoping that the client will not notice!

Hygiene Wash hands before and after treatments using an antibacterial agent and maintain a high level of cleanliness in the massage environment.

First aid for therapists

A basic knowledge of first aid is a must for anyone practising massage and is useful to have, even as a student, as a treatment may provoke some reaction that requires your attention. Your insurance company and professional association will require you to hold a first-aid qualification, as will any potential employer when applying for jobs.

Clients will feel reassured that the person treating them is qualified to deal with medical emergencies and if you are thinking of running your own clinic an appointed person trained in health and safety first aid is a legal requirement.

Even if you are a qualified first aider, it will be necessary to update your training every three years as views change on how to deal with emergencies. For example, the correct 'recovery position' is quite different from what was thought to be suitable a few years ago.

A basic course is generally only one day in duration and covers the following topics:

- principles of first aid at work
- cardiopulmonary resuscitation (CPR)
- control of bleeding
- burns and scalds
- duties of first-aid appointed persons, including simple record keeping
- first-aid kits/box contents and use of
- emergency resuscitation
- external chest compressions
- electrical injuries
- care of the unconscious patient
- other medical emergencies, including angina attacks, asthma attacks, choking, eye injuries, fainting, fractures, seizures, hypoglycaemia, poisoning, severe allergic reaction, shock.

Perhaps the most useful knowledge gleaned on a course is recovery positions and what to do if a client has an asthma attack or becomes hypoglycaemic. The following guidelines can act as a reminder and are no substitute for training from a professional first aid instructor.

The recovery position

If a client loses consciousness or becomes very light-headed then they need to be placed in a safe position for the recovery process. The position will be different depending on their age or if injury has occurred.

For a baby up to 12 months of age, call for medical help immediately. Cradle the baby in your arms, with the head tilted downwards to prevent choking on the tongue or inhaling any vomit. Monitor and record vital signs, for example the level of their response, pulse and breathing.

For a child or adult over the age of one year, if the person is unconscious but has no other obvious life-threatening conditions place them in the recovery position as follows:

1 Turn the person onto their side.
2 Lift chin forward in open airway position and adjust hand under the cheek as necessary.
3 Check they cannot roll forwards or backwards.
4 Monitor breathing and pulse continuously.
5 Turn to the other side after 30 minutes.

If there is a possibility of spinal injury, take care not to tilt the neck, place your hands on either side of their face and with your fingertips gently lift the jaw to open the airway.

Asthma attack

During an asthma attack the muscles of the air passages go into spasm, the linings of the airways swell and breathing becomes difficult as the passageways narrow. These attacks can be triggered by allergy, the cold, smoke or extremes in temperature. Clients with asthma usually deal well with their own attacks by using a blue reliever inhaler, but there may be occasions where you are required to assist.

A person having asthma attack is likely to display the following:

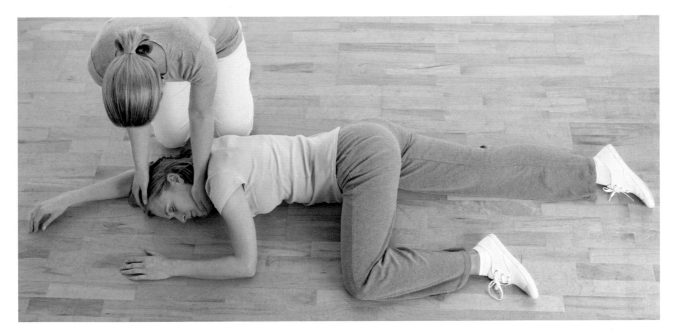

- Wheezing when breathing out.
- Difficulty in breathing, with a very prolonged breathing-out phase.
- Difficulty speaking and whispering.
- Distress and anxiety.
- Coughing.
- Features of hypoxia, such as a grey-blue tinge to the lips, earlobes and nailbeds (cyanosis).

The aim during an asthma attack is to ease the breathing and call for medical help if necessary. Make sure your client is sitting, do not let them lie down. Keep them calm and encourage them to breathe slowly and deeply.

Caution: If this is the first attack, or if the attack is severe and any one of the following occurs:
- The inhaler has no effect after five minutes.
- The client becomes worse.
- Breathlessness makes talking difficult.
- The client becomes exhausted.

Call for an ambulance and whilst waiting for its arrival encourage the client to use their inhaler every five to ten minutes. Monitor their breathing and pulse and record to inform the paramedics on arrival.

If the client becomes unconscious, open their airway, check their breathing and be ready to give emergency aid.

Hypoglycaemia (low blood sugar)

When blood sugar levels fall below normal the brain function is affected, sometimes recognized by a rapidly deteriorating level of response. This generally occurs in

Recovery position The recovery position shown above is for adults. Different criteria will apply for babies under one year old or where spinal injury is a possibility.

people with diabetes and on rare occasions after a session of binge drinking. The features to look out for are:

- Palpitations and muscle tremors, although the pulse may be strong.
- Weakness, faintness or hunger.
- Strange actions or behaviour.
- Sweating and cold, clammy skin.
- Deteriorating level of response.

The aim of treatment is to raise the blood sugar content as quickly as possible and call for medical help if necessary. If the client is already on the massage table they should remain lying down. If not on the table assist them to sit or lie down. Give them a sugary drink, sugar lumps or other sweet food (e.g. chocolate). DO NOT administer diet drinks as they do not contain the sugar needed. Advise them to see their doctor even if fully recovered.

Warning: If consciousness is impaired do not give them anything to eat or drink in case they are not able to swallow or drink it properly.

If the client loses consciousness, open their airway and check breathing; if normal, place in the recovery position and call for an ambulance. If they stop breathing, give chest compressions and rescue breaths.

Working positions

Whether you are working on a massage table, chair or floormat, your posture and positioning plays an important part in the continuity, rhythm and flow of the treatment.

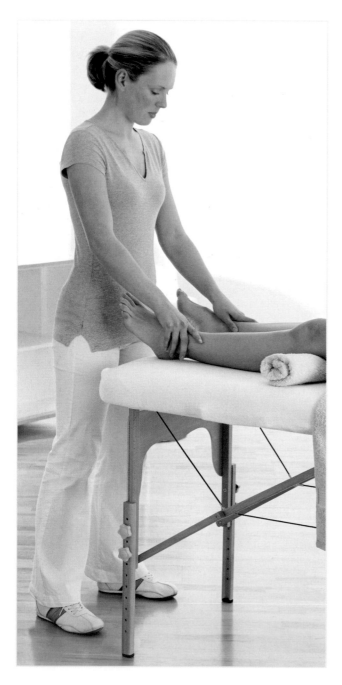

Massage dictates that you move from a stable base and that the pressure you apply transmits from the stability of the lower body, the position of the feet influencing the direction and type of stroke being applied.

The main rules for working with a massage table are to stand square to the table, bend from your knees and hips and do not twist your body. Always move backwards and forwards and side to side using three main postures: upright, warrior and monkey or tai chi position.

Working with the client seated will involve a combination of the upright and warrior stances. When working on the floor, similar positions are used but from a kneeling, rather than standing position, making sure the back remains straight and when stretching forward, lifting up from the knees slightly in order not to round or arch the back.

Upright position

Standing with your back straight and feet slightly apart, balance your body weight equally on both legs. The pressure should be directed through the arms, not the wrist to point of contact. Usually parallel to the table you can lean forward slightly without tensing the back muscles by tilting the pelvis. This position is often used when working side-on to the table and applying strokes to the opposite side of the client's body – stretching to the other side of the table. It is also the position for some techniques at the head or foot of the table, when applying massage to the head, face, shoulders and feet.

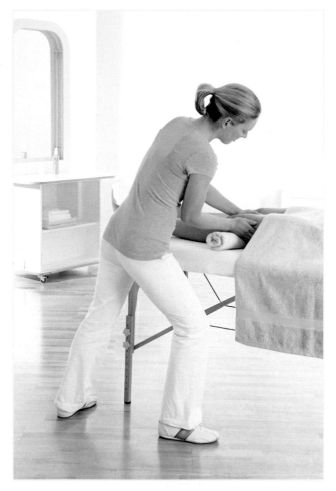

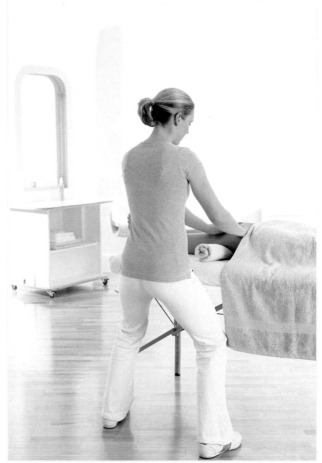

Warrior position

Sometimes called the lunge, this position has your legs parallel, but with one foot ahead of the other, toes facing forwards. The further apart you place the feet, the stronger the stroke will be. As you lean forward, apply the pressure through the arms to the point of contact, using your bodyweight behind the stroke by raising the heel of the back foot slightly, at the same time keeping the front leg relaxed. Arms should be straight or slightly flexed at the elbow and your back straight.

If working with one hand, your massage arm can be slightly flexed at the elbow while the other arm is held straight and placed in a suitable position to maintain contact with your client.

Working at either end of the table or side-on, this position allows you to determine the pressure of the stroke. The movement is backwards and forwards as the weight is shifted from foot to foot, forwards for the upwards strokes and backwards for the return strokes. It is used when applying any long strokes, as in effleurage, or that travel along the client's body.

Monkey position

The monkey or tai chi position is similar to a plié in ballet. Standing a little way from the edge of the table but parallel to it, with your back upright and arms straight, place your body weight equally over both feet, with the knees slightly flexed. Shift your weight side to side in a movement that can be slight or exaggerated, depending on the manoeuvre required. A slight rotation of the trunk can also exert a gentle pulling action with the arm. The monkey position with legs straight rather than slightly flexed is called the upright position and is used for applying strokes travelling relatively short distances such as petrissage or friction.

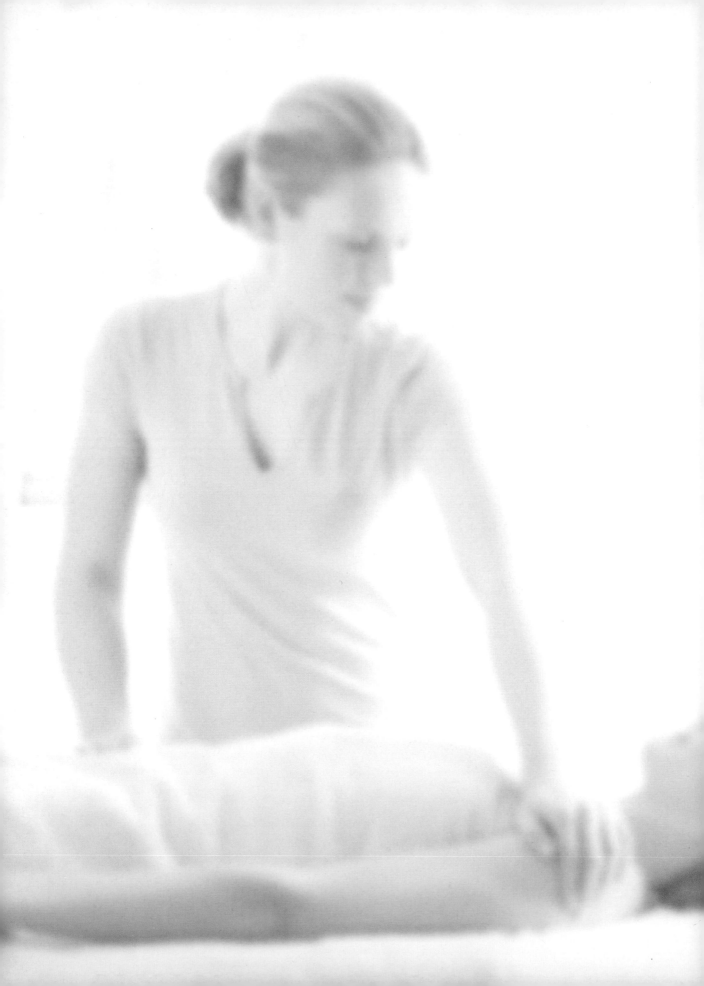

Massage techniques

In the Western world the most widely used system of massage is based on basic strokes: effleurage, petrissage, friction and percussion. A massage routine starts with some movements to establish initial contact and ends with connecting or 'grounding' holds. Mastery of these basic movements, combined with communication and awareness skills, equip a therapist with the means to develop and adapt their massage.

Introduction to massage

Massage is much more than just manipulation of the soft tissue; a skilful therapist uses their own body mechanics, together with pressure, depth and direction of strokes that are applied with continuity and rhythm at various speeds and duration.

Each massage session is unique as the response from the client changes according to the application. As a student your concentration will be on remembering the strokes and their order, but with practice these will become second nature. Once you are qualified, you can shift the emphasis onto adapting this basic knowledge, even creating your own techniques.

Pressure and depth

Your hands act as sensors to the responses of the soft tissue manipulations and so your client's body will be your road map and direct the session. Pressure is the force with which a massage stroke is applied and depth is how far it travels into the soft tissue. As a therapist you will use your body weight channelled through your arms to apply pressure with your hands, forearms or elbows. Occasionally hand-held massage tools designed for specific purposes may be introduced. In Eastern massage techniques, pressure is often applied with the knees and feet instead of hands. These movements can be integrated into a regular massage routine where appropriate.

The amount of pressure and depth you use will depend on the state of the muscle you are working on. A relaxed muscle will allow you to work deeply, whereas one holding tension will be guarded and will only react to lighter touch. In general, a massage session will begin with light pressured stokes, gradually building up the pressure to a level the client is comfortable with.

Stroke direction and rhythm

The direction of the strokes depends on their type. Effleurage, for example, is generally applied in a downwards and forwards direction, whereas friction work may employ circular or back and forth movement. The distance travelled will depend on whether you want to work the whole length of a muscle or stay focused on a specific area.

Rhythm, continuity, and the way the massage is delivered is very important in gaining your clients' confidence and helping them relax. A treatment needs to flow with smooth transition from one stroke to another, maintaining contact at all time. The speed and rhythm of execution will alter to suit the reason for the massage: slow for a client requiring relaxation or faster where stimulation is required. You may decide to change these elements within a single treatment to achieve the outcome desired, while maintaining continuity. It is important to remember that working too fast or too slow can reduce the effectiveness of your strokes.

Duration

The decision on the amount of time or duration spent massaging an area will be something that will become clearer as you gain experience. The client will not show signs of overwork until much later or even the following day, when they may complain of a tenderness similar to that caused by slight sunburn. This is the muscle's response to excessive deep-tissue massage by becoming slightly inflamed and application of an ice pack or cooling gel will reduce the symptoms. Do not be tempted to over focus on a problem area, in remedial massage often 'more is less'.

Warming up

A massage therapist needs to be relaxed and flexible when giving a treatment, as each move or tension, however slight, is magnified when transferred through contact to the client.

Preparation by the use of a simple routine of self-massage and stretching will improve the physical strength and stamina required to give a massage treatment. It will help regulate breathing patterns and focus your mind. Your own body mechanics and the way you apply your massage will benefit from warming up and clearing the mind.

The following self-massage routines are performed sitting down with the arms supported at a comfortable height for the strokes to deliver the most effect.

Self-massage

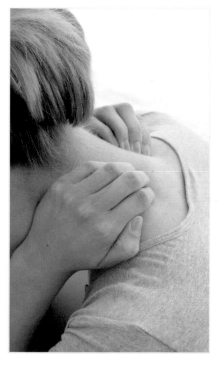 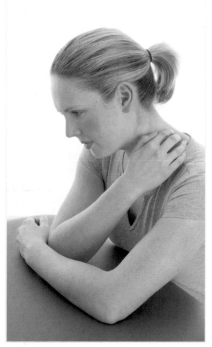 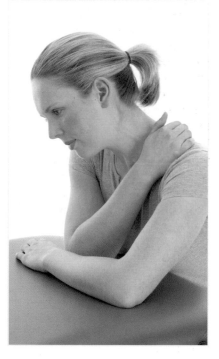

1 In a seated position, resting your elbows on a table or other flat surface, lean forward and place your hands at the back of your neck behind each ear, inclining your head slightly forward. Using only the pads of the fingers make small circles, applying pressure at the same time, and work along the neck either side of the spine.

2 Keeping your left hand on the table, place your right hand on your left shoulder and slowly squeeze the muscle between your fingers and the heel of your hand, tilting your head away from the area you are massaging. Work outwards from the base of the neck to the edge of the shoulder.

3 Repeat, but this time instead of squeezing the muscle, apply pressure through the pads of the fingers in small circular movements as before. Place the hand back on the table and repeat the whole sequence on the opposite side.

Warming up *continued*

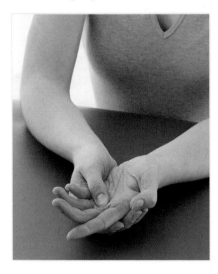

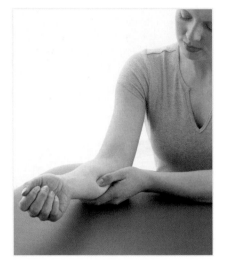

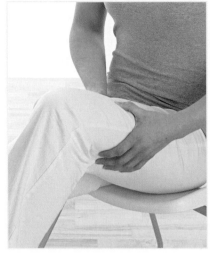

4 With palms upwards, place your right hand under your left hand for support with the right thumb resting on the left palm. Using the pad of the thumb, apply slow circular strokes with deep pressure, moving over the whole hand, including the fingers. Change hands and repeat the sequence.

5 Resting one hand on the table, support the arm with the fingers of the opposite hand, and using the thumb pad as before, apply pressure through slow circular strokes up the forearm, from the wrist to the elbow. Where you may feel pockets of tension, work the area until the muscle releases any tightness.

6 If your legs are feeling tired, remain seated and rest the ankle of the leg you want to work on the opposite knee or a stool. Place webbed hands either side of the thigh, with the thumbs resting on the top, then use the pads to make deep circular strokes as before. Move over the whole thigh and back of the calf, paying extra attention to any areas of tension. When finished, smooth over the whole area with the flat of your hand before changing legs and repeating the sequence.

Stretches

The next set of stretches are performed standing up and can be added at the end of the self-massage routine or used alone just prior to or between massage sessions.

1 Warm your hands by placing them together in a prayer position and briskly rub them up and down against each other. Using the right hand, rub the back of the left hand, working over the wrist and up the arm before changing hands to warm the opposite side.

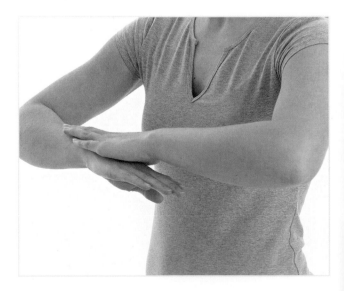

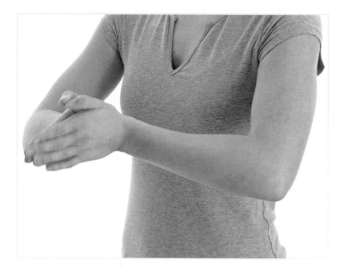

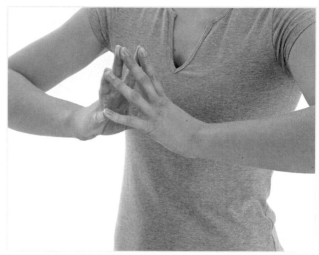

2 Return your hands to the prayer position holding them at chest level, then rotate your forearms and wrists so that the hands move up and down in a quick movement, repeating several times.

3 Keeping your hands in same position, open your wrists until they are 13–15cm (5–6in) apart by pressing the pads of the fingers together, at the same time spreading the fingers wide. Once you have reached your natural extension release the pressure, returning to the start position in order to repeat several times.

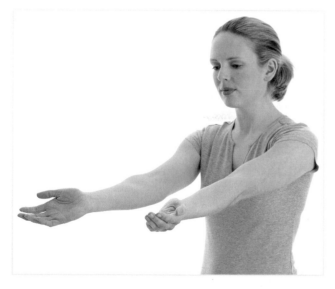

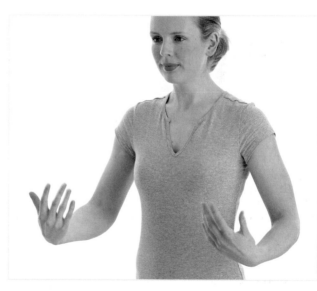

4 Stretch out both arms in front of you at chest level and circle both hands clockwise for eight to ten revolutions; repeating in an anti-clockwise direction. Next, make both hands into fists and repeat the sequence.

5 Using a wrist action, shake both hands and fingers vigorously. Finish by dropping your arms to your sides, ready to rotate your shoulders first forwards and then backwards, repeating five to ten times each way.

To finish

When you are adequately warmed up, stand still, taking two or three long, deep breaths, exhaling slowly. Now you are well prepared to apply your massage techniques.

Effleurage

Originating from a French word meaning 'stroking' or 'to glide', effleurage is one of the classic massage techniques and probably the first one you will learn. It can be used everywhere on the body and is a sweeping, rhythmic stroke that is used at the beginning and end of a massage treatment to make and break contact.

Effleurage allows the therapist to sense areas of tension and also to spread massage oil, lotion, cream, wax or powder. It warms the muscles in preparation for deeper work and allows the recipient to relax and adjust to the therapist's touch.

Effleurage also promotes the flow of blood and lymph, induces relaxation and is the main stroke used to bring out the aromatherapeutic benefits of essential oils. It is the most commonly applied Swedish stroke as it used to connect different sections of a massage treatment.

Flat-handed effleurage
After oiling the flats of your hands, make contact with your client, keeping your wrists relaxed and fingers together.

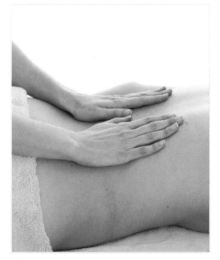 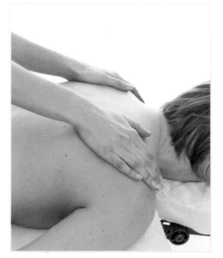 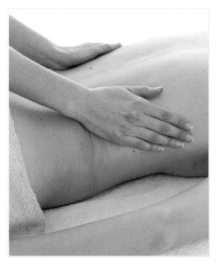

1 Glide both hands simultaneously alongside each other, working away from yourself to your natural reach, applying pressure at the same time.

2 Maintaining contact, separate and return the stroke in a breaststroke-like movement. Mould your hands into the contours of the client's body and build the upward pressure on each stroke. Pressure should be on the upward stroke with only the weight of the hands on return, the deeper the upward stroke, the slower it should be applied.

3 When working on the back, remember to place your hands either side of the spine and do not work directly over it. When gliding over joint areas, lift off any pressure, still maintaining contact.

Double-handed or reinforced effleurage

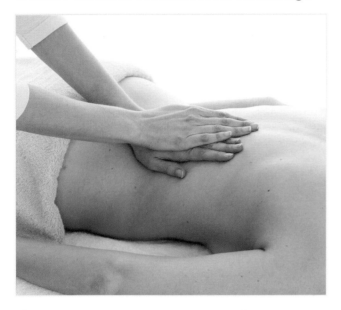

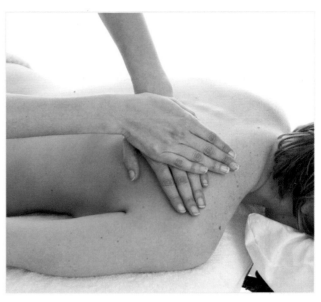

1 Place one hand on top of the other to reinforce the stroke. This is useful where deeper pressure is required or when working on specific areas.

2 Double-handed effleurage can also be applied in a circular movement, which is useful when working the shoulder and stomach areas.

One-handed effleurage

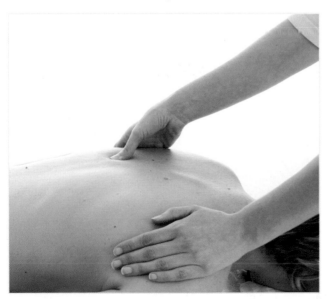

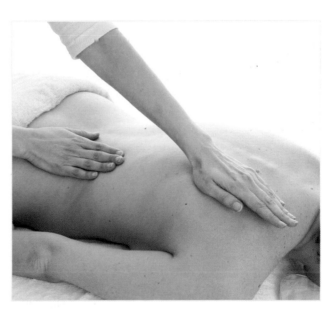

1 Apply only one hand or one thumb pad at a time. This is useful when focusing on small areas such as the metatarsals or the neck and shoulder along the trapezius.

2 You can also apply the stroke with alternate hands or thumbs. Glide one hand upwards and at the end of the upward stroke lift off, ensuring at the same time the alternate hand starts the next stroke, repeating the movement and maintaining contact.

Cupped effleurage

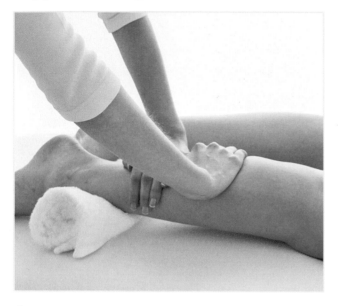

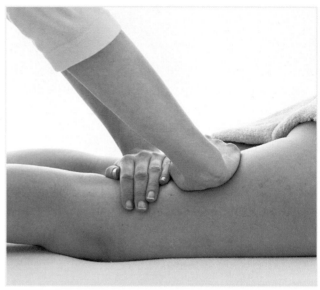

1 For this variation, place the oiled hands horizontally one above the other and slightly cupped. This is particularly useful when working on arms or legs.

2 As with flat-handed effleurage, glide up the limb with cupped hands to your natural reach, turn and use the flat-handed stroke to return.

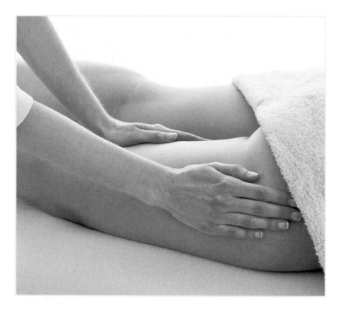

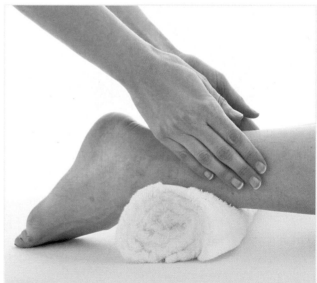

3 When working the upper leg, take the stroke further, with the outside hand into the gluteals whilst discreetly turning the hand on the inner thigh so as not to be intrusive.

4 All styles of effleurage can be used in reverse, keeping pressure as always on the upward stroke, to work the soft tissue in a different way. Self-care: avoid any hypertension of your wrist. The angle that you work at should be approximately 100–180 degrees, and hands, arms, torso and legs should all follow the path of movement in alignment. Also make sure your thumb is tucked in against the forefinger.

Petrissage

Derived from the French word *petrir*, 'to knead' or 'to mash', petrissage is the general name given to any strokes that squeeze, press or roll the soft tissue, working parallel to the muscle fibres. It is similar to the kneading process in breadmaking and usually follows the effleurage strokes, preparing for deeper work such as friction.

Petrissage 'milks' the muscles of metabolic waste, promotes blood and oxygen return to the tissues and relaxes the muscles by stretching and loosening the fascia.

Two-handed petrissage

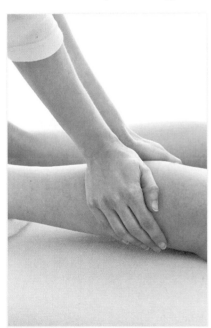 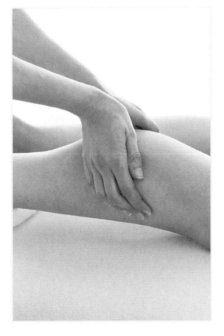 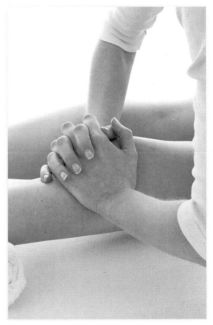

1 Make contact with your hands on the top of the muscle, at the same time using your fingertips to support the underside in a C shape.

2 Each hand mirroring the other, raise the muscle and skin away from the bone. With the heel of the hand, compress the tissue downwards, lifting off the pressure, ready to repeat the rhythmical pattern of lifting, squeezing and releasing. Work over the whole of the muscle area before moving to another.

3 A variation on this when working legs and arms is to place the hands in the opposite position over the muscle, by interlacing the fingers in a prayer like position on top of the muscle. Use the heel of the hand to lift, squeeze and release.

Alternate-hand petrissage

This technique can also be applied using each hand alternatively rather than simultaneously.

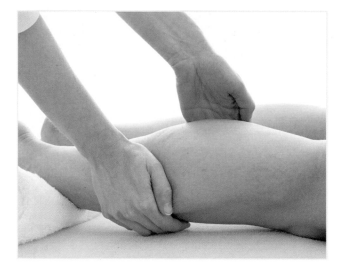

With one hand, compress the tissue downwards whilst the other hand is lifting and stretching upwards, making sure that contact is maintained. This is useful to apply over larger areas, such as the side of the buttocks, working one side at a time, side-on.

One-handed petrissage

This is used most effectively when strong pressure is required or when working in smaller areas, such as along the trapezius or the back, either side of the spine.

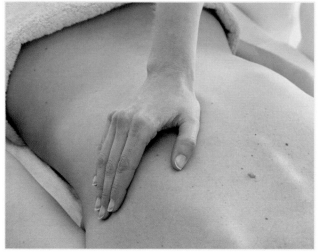

Keeping one hand resting on the limb or torso, use the other to apply the petrissage stroke, working over the muscle area and adjusting the pressure according to the tension. In the case of infant massage, using one hand the tissue is manipulated between the pads of the fingers and thumb.

Kneading

Sometimes this stroke is thought of as the only petrissage stroke. It is applied with medium pressure, only after the muscle has been relaxed and is most beneficial over large, fleshy areas with slow, deep strokes. Unlike effleurage, the whole hand with thumbs spread is employed in this side-to-side action.

An alternative method of kneading is to place the hands either side of the muscle to be worked with the thumbs linked and crossed on the top of the area. The tissue is squeezed and rolled in a circular motion.

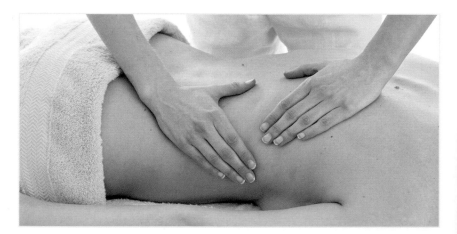

Place both hands next to each other over the area to be worked, making a 'C' shape between the fingers and thumb. Lean into the muscle and, using one hand first, squeeze and roll the muscle. Repeat the move with the other hand. Kneading should be a continuous, rhythmic motion that can vary in speed as required. As with other methods of petrissage, the stroke can also be applied with one hand, using either the whole of the hand or the finger and thumb pads, whichever is appropriate for the area being worked.

Pulling

This is a simple technique to perform but it is very effective. Once the muscles have been loosened, apply this stroke to lift the muscles away from the bone using the flats of the fingers and holding the position for a few seconds before releasing. This will aid relaxation and release of tension. There are two easy areas to introduce this into a massage routine, the first whilst working on the side of the torso and the second on the back.

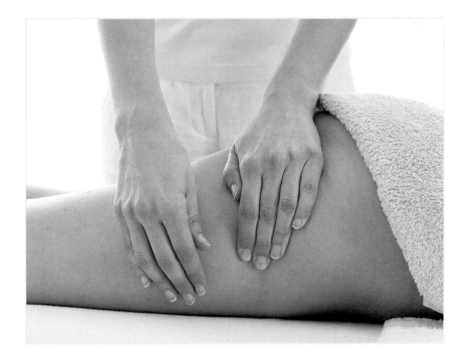

1 Whilst working side-on to the client, start at the gluteal area and with both hands side by side, use the flat of the fingers to pull the muscle slowly and firmly, holding for a couple of seconds before releasing. Use this technique to work the length of the side of the torso and return, before moving to the other side. The stroke can also be applied with alternate hands, as the first hand finishes the motion the other starts.

2 Having applied effleurage and petrissage on the back and shoulders, slide hands over the shoulders, one hand on each side and hook the flat and pads of the fingers into the muscles at the front of the shoulders. Using your body weight for maximum effect, lift up and pull back both sides simultaneously, holding for a few seconds before releasing and repeating two or three times.

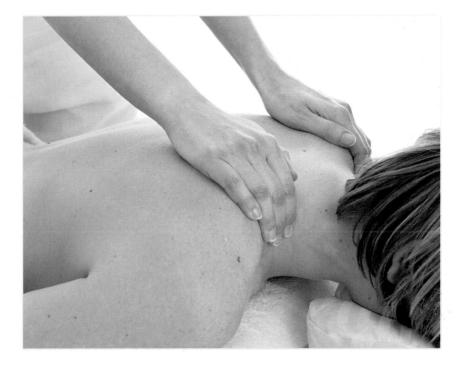

Squeezing

Sometimes known as skin rolling, this stroke also plays a major role in other bodywork techniques such as myofascial release. Before using this technique, which works on the superficial fascia, remove any excess oil or other lubricant.

1 Using fingers and thumbs, grasp and lift the skin, at the same time compressing the soft tissue. Slowly move across the desired area, using your fingers to move and gather the tissue to be worked on.

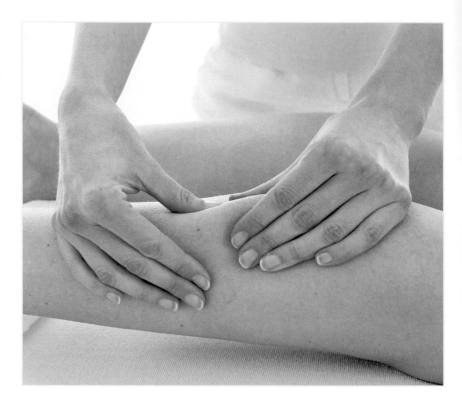

2 Lift and roll the fascia in different directions as the fascia also lies in different planes. To do this you can lift the skin between the sides of your two hands lying flat over an area or by bringing the thumb web of one hand towards the tops of the fingers of the other in a 'T' shape. Whichever position you employ, do not force the tissue.

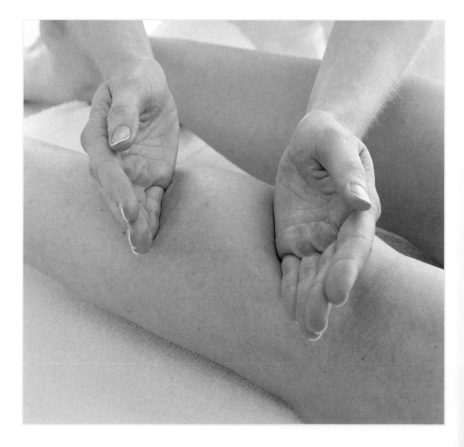

Wringing

This stroke is so named because it aims to 'wring' out the tension and metabolic waste that may be stored in the muscle.

Using the whole of the hand with the thumbs closed to the fingers, work alternatively backwards and forwards over the area, lifting the skin towards you with one hand whilst pushing away with the other. Open the thumbs wide when working on smaller muscles in order to stabilize your grip as you wring. Pressure should be even and as there is no downward compression, the stroke may be used with care over bonier areas. Wringing is often applied on the calf, thigh and lower back areas. Combining squeezing and lifting, wringing is a useful stroke to link others in a massage sequence.

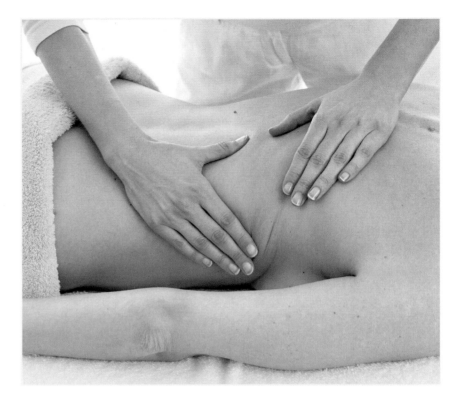

Opening

Sometimes called pulling petrissage or broadening, this stroke opens out the muscle and other soft tissue around the bone, rather similar to a contracting muscle.

It is possible to apply this stroke with one hand by using the fingers to pull the tissue up towards the heel of the hand in order to then apply pressure, resulting in the skin rolling forward and stretching the underlying muscle fibres. Once the heel of the hand reaches the fingers, release and reposition to repeat the stroke once the tissues have returned to their normal position. This stroke is very effective on the deltoid, trapezius and scapula muscles.

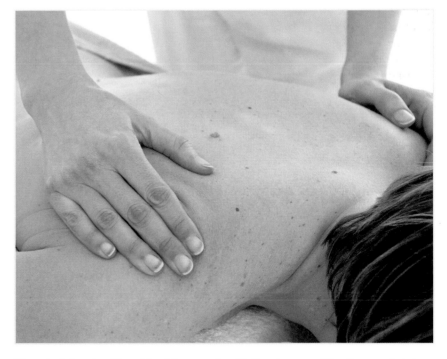

Place both hands either side of the muscle with thumbs open. Simultaneously bring the thumbs in towards the fingers, lifting the tissue up and away from the bone at the same time spreading and stretching the muscle.

Friction

Derived from the Latin word *frictio*, 'to rub', friction strokes are deep, focused strokes that follow effleurage and petrissage in a massage routine.

Performed by rubbing one surface over the other using mainly fingertips, thumbs and heel of hands, friction can be applied both deeply and superficially. In deep-friction work the action is not of gliding over the skin but of moving the skin and fascia across the soft tissue, compressing it against the bone. It is usually applied without the use of a lubricant. The movements are classified as rubbing, rolling, circling, cross-fibre and parallel friction. These strokes stimulate circulation and light friction can be used to reduce oedema, disperse calcifications around joint areas and release and stretch knots of tension. Care should be taken not to exacerbate any area where the nerve is inflamed or that reacts protectively to touch.

Rubbing

Sometimes known as heat rub, this superficial friction technique is usually applied to the larger areas of the back or arms. If applied with the edge of the hands it is known as 'sawing' and 'towel' friction is where a towel is introduced as a massage tool. Rubbing is the most instinctive of massage techniques, used in everyday life.

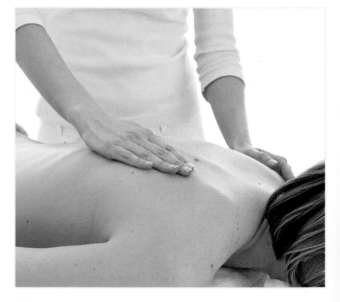

1 Using both hands palm down with thumbs and fingers closed together, make contact and, using a brisk motion, move the hands simultaneously in opposite directions to the outer edges of the area being treated.

2 Return, with the hands passing each other in midstroke. Continue this back and forth motion, increasing speed until the area is warmed. You can also adapt this to work over suitable areas by rubbing with one hand, applying pressure in a circular motion whilst the other hand maintains contact. If the area to be worked is small, the finger pads or knuckles can be used to apply the strokes rather than the full flat of the hand, to achieve the same results.

Rolling

Thumb rolling uses the full length of your thumbs, keeping the rest of the hand in contact.

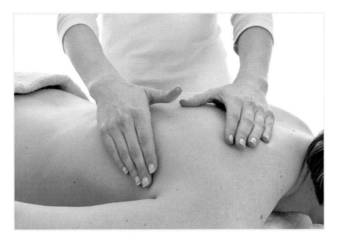

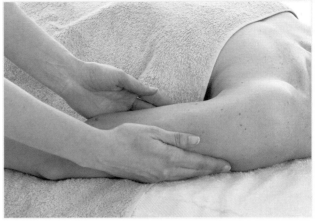

1 Bring one thumb down behind the other, pushing away with short, deep strokes, compressing the soft tissue in a rhythmic motion. This is useful when focusing on both small and large areas, smoothing out pockets of tension as you identify them. The area between the spine and scapula responds particularly well to this type of friction.

2 Other rolling strokes are used when working on the legs and arms. If the client is supine, ask them to extend the limb, then take it between the palms of both extended hands and, moving in opposite directions, roll the skin, soft tissue and muscle around the bone, applying pressure at the same time. You can apply this stroke working up the extremity, sliding your hands from distal to proximal positions.

Heel of hand

Using the heel of the hands allows you to apply firm pressure, pushing forwards firmly into the soft tissue.

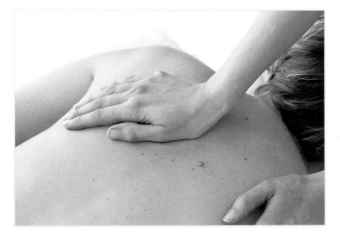

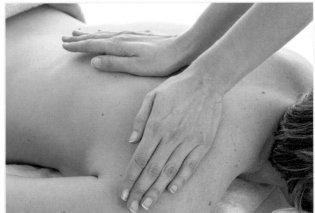

1 Working with alternate hands, make contact with the heel of one hand, followed shortly by the other in a continuous rhythm across the muscle area.

2 When working on the scapula area, make contact with the both hands, fingers held lightly in position, apply pressure through the heels of the hand whilst at the same time pushing slightly upwards and outwards, your left hand moving anti-clockwise whilst the right hand moves clockwise. This can also be applied one hand at a time, the other maintaining contact.

Circling

For small areas, work with one hand, keeping contact with the other.

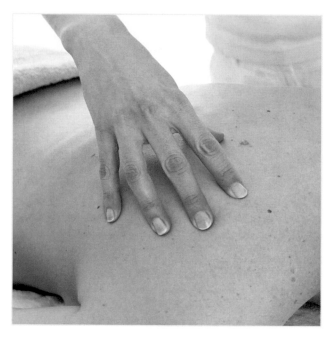

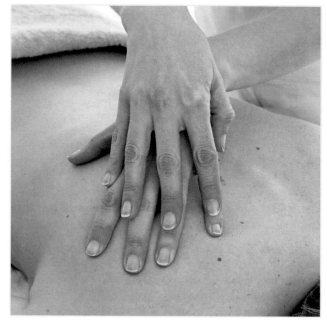

1 Move your fingers slightly apart and using the pads apply even pressure, at the same time moving over the soft tissue in very small circular motions. Start with gentle pressure, increasing slowly as you work over the area.

2 Deep-friction circling is applied by placing one hand on top of the other, keeping the fingers straight but relaxed. Make contact with the finger pads only and lean into the muscle, using small circular motions to work the area. If working around the knee joint, substitute the finger pads with a single thumb pad.

3 The knuckles can also be used by curling your hands into a loose fist and rotating the hand at the same time as applying pressure through the knuckles. An adaptation of this stroke is to rotate the fingers at the same time as making the circular movement. This is great for working the backs of the hands and the top of the foot. Tension often found around the pectoral muscles or the scapula responds well to circular knuckling and clients usually find it very pleasant to receive.

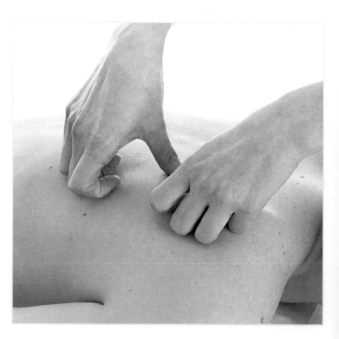

Cross-fibre friction

This is sometimes referred to as deep transverse friction. It is very focused and used often in sports and remedial treatments. In order to apply this stroke you need to have good knowledge of muscle-fibre patterns and be able to identify the areas of tension.

Placing the thumb or finger pads at the exact site of the tension or pain, use a back and forth motion in a direction across the fibres, applying even pressure and making sure that you do not drag the skin. The amount of pressure will depend on the client's tolerance level and should only be applied for 10–15 seconds at a time. Tensions and adhesions of the muscles, ligaments and tendons respond well to cross-fibre friction.

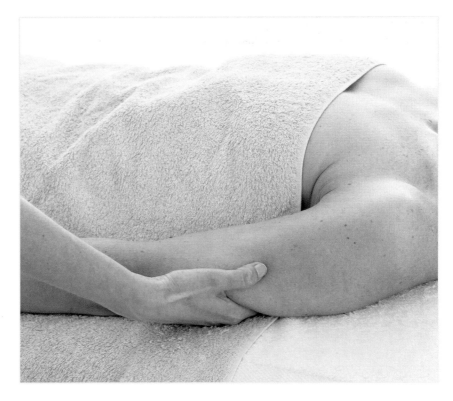

Parallel friction

As with the cross-fibre stroke, parallel friction requires good knowledge of the muscle-fibre patterns as you work along rather than across the lay of the muscles, tendons and ligaments.

Parallel friction is also useful in addressing the soft tissue between very bony areas such as the metacarpals and metatarsals and the lower arms and legs.

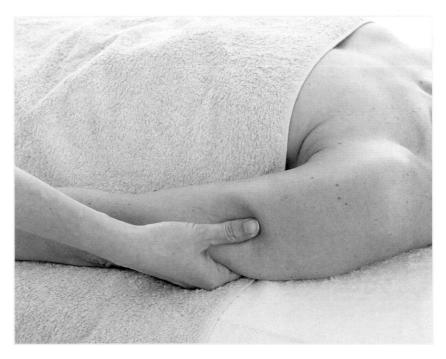

Apply the stroke with one hand, maintaining contact and support with the other. This is a versatile stroke: you can use thumb, finger pads or knuckles, working in a simple backwards and forwards rubbing motion.

Percussion or tapotement

Known as either percussion from the Latin *percutere*, 'to hit', or tapotement, from the French word *taper*, meaning a 'light blow', this technique incorporates strokes that involve repetitive light striking movements, applied briskly and rhythmically with a certain amount of noise.

Variations of percussion are classified as tapping, pinching, hacking, cupping, pounding and clapping. Their are used depends on the area being treated and the effect you are trying to receive.

The pressure of the strokes should be adjusted according to where they are applied. Delicate or thin tissued areas require lighter touch than muscular areas. Do not apply percussion over the lower back area above the kidneys as there is not enough tissue protection from these forceful strokes.

Unlike some other techniques, percussion can be applied both directly or through towels or clothing and is often used as a 'wake up' stroke towards the end of a treatment or when finishing a specific area. During an invigorating massage, percussion is used to stimulate the body's systems and increase circulation to localized areas.

Percussive strokes should be executed with loose and relaxed wrists and fingers, allowing the hands to spring back after contact. This enables you to control the force, speed and smoothness of the stroke.

Tapping

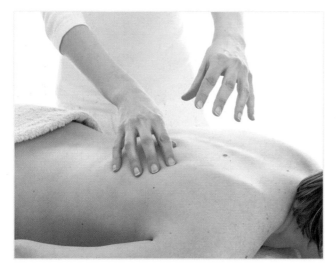

1 Using the fingertips of both hands, make contact by striking the client's body with a consistent speed and pressure, lifting off one hand and applying the other alternatively. For a different effect, use one hand only, alternating the pressure between light and deep with each strike. Raindrops is a term often used when tapping is applied to the face or scalp, the desired effect is that of light rain, hence the name.

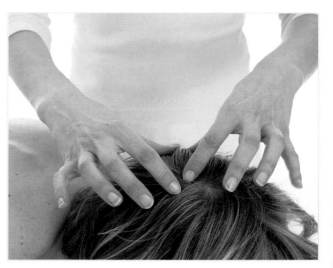

2 Using all ten finger pads at the same time, very lightly 'drum' the surface of the skin, each fingertip striking at a different time, one after the other. This technique can also be used gently on the scalp.

Cupping

Cupping is often used in a clinical setting to help loosen mucus or phlegm held in the chest. The client should have the abdomen and chest raised by extra bolsters or pillows so that the head is in a lower position, and the therapist should be ready to pause during the technique, with tissues to hand. The cupping may induce coughing, which is a good sign that the residues are loosening. Any discomfort experienced can be relieved with the application of soothing effleurage at the end of the procedure.

Form a cup with each hand and use the same motion as hacking, the edge of the 'cups' making contact, with alternate strikes. The vacuum created causes a hollow suction sound when the hand is lifted off. This suction stimulates circulation and some localized redness may be visible.

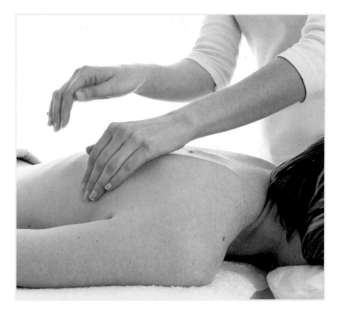

Hacking

Probably the most well known of percussive strokes, this 'chopping' motion is synonymous with classical Swedish massage. The stroke is applied with the ulnar edge of each hand.

Hacking along muscle fibre will help break down any tension being held and relax the muscle.

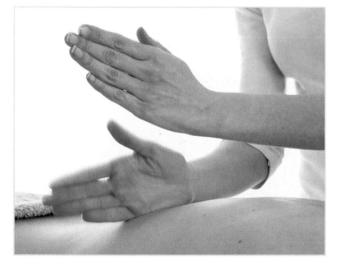

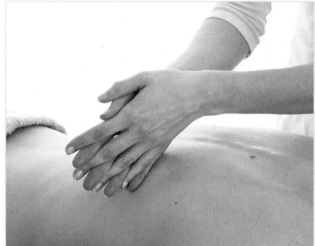

1 With fingers held slightly apart and wrists loose, apply the stroke with alternate hands. As the hand strikes the body, the vibration causes each finger to make contact with the one above it, so strokes should be kept light and relaxed to avoid any repetitive strain injuries.

2 An alternative version of hacking, useful for working on areas such as the rhomboids, is to place your hands together, fingers held slightly apart and to strike with the sides of the last three fingers rather than the whole side of the hands.

Pinching

Sometimes known as pincement or plucking, the motion is similar to tapping.

Using hands alternatively, grasp the top of the skin between the thumb and finger pads and lift slightly before releasing. The aim is to slightly lift the skin as in petrissage strokes and not to pinch or bruise, whilst maintaining a regular rhythm.

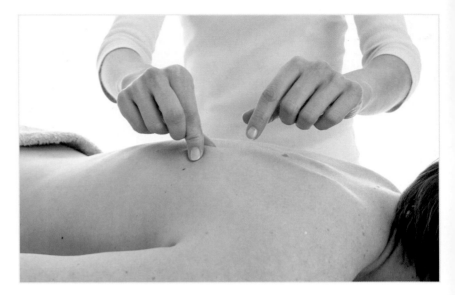

Pounding

Pounding, or pummeling as it is sometimes called, should only be used over muscular areas with good protective layers such as the posterior thigh and gluteal regions.

Using a similar motion to the hacking stroke but with the hands formed into loose fists, make contact with the side of the fist, applying moderate pressure. An alternative version is to strike with the knuckles facing downwards, rather similar to knocking at a door.

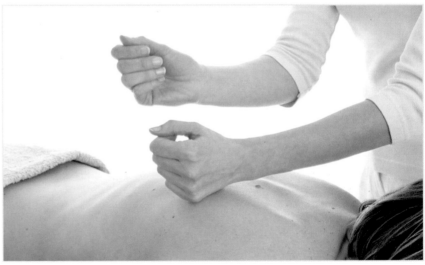

Clapping

Clapping is sometimes referred to as slapping. It helps stimulate nerve endings and bring tone to flaccid muscles. It may not be suitable for use where a client associates this type of stroke with negative experiences.

With a flat hand, use the palm and flats of the fingers to strike the surface of the skin alternatively and rhythmically. This is like the cupping stroke applied with the flat of the hand. The pressure should be very light and can even be applied to the sides of the face with care.

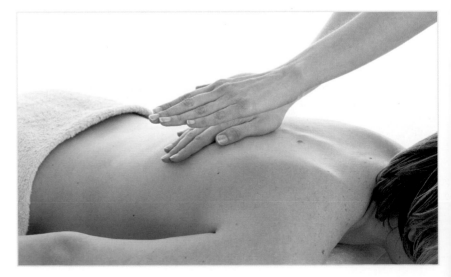

Other techniques

Various other techniques, such as feathering, raking, vibration, joint mobilization and passive stretching can be added to the four major massage strokes to make up a complete routine.

Feathering

Sometimes considered a type of effleurage stroke, feathering is a gentle gliding of the fingertips over the skin. Pressure should be featherweight and consistent for this technique, which is used to relax and often applied as a finishing stroke.

Raking

This is another light stroke that could be considered a type of effleurage. Raking is a connecting stroke that allows the therapist to move from one side of the table to the other whilst maintaining contact.

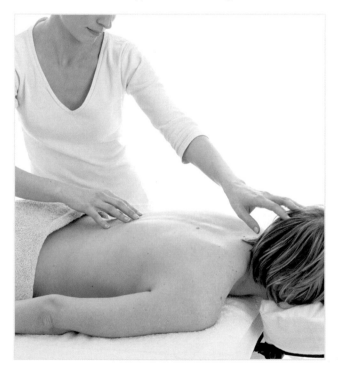

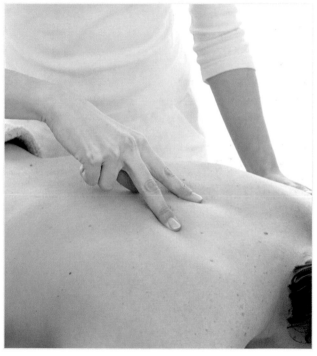

With the hands flat and fingers slightly apart, apply the stroke with the fingertips up the length of the muscle, working toward you with one hand, followed by the other. Use one hand whilst maintaining contact with the other. When the fingertips reach the end of the muscle length, instead of lifting off, turn the hand over and work back along the muscle, using the fronts of the fingers in a combing movement. Make sure that the up stroke and return are executed in one flowing sweep, using either light or firm pressure, whichever is required.

Form a V shape with the index and middle fingers of one hand and place the fingertips either side of the spine. Pull down a section of the muscles, one hand after the other until the whole area is worked.

Vibration

From the Latin *vibrare*, vibration is a shaking or rocking movement applied both mechanically and manually using the fingertips or the full hand.

To achieve fine vibrations, only the fingertips are used to 'tremble' the tissue by moving them rapidly up and down or side to side.

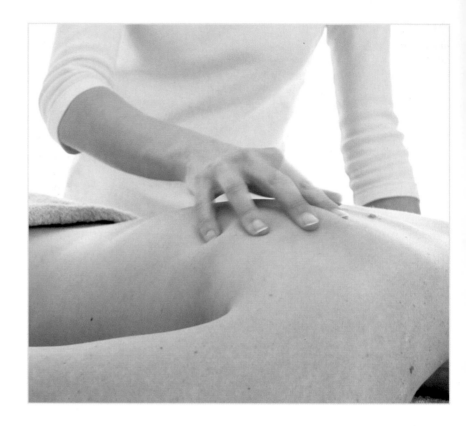

Rocking

This uses both hands in a movement that involves pushing the client's body back and forth between the two hands, working with its natural rhythm, not fighting it. This can be physically demanding on the therapist but very soothing for the client.

Rocking is applied at the beginning of a routine or area being worked where there is much tension held. The muscle is literally rocked and unlocked. It is also a simple way of relaxing the client and familiarizing them with your touch.

Take the part of the body that needs working between the flats of both hands. With firm contact, push between one hand and the other until it swings relaxed between the two. When working on the torso, use hand-over-hand contact to rock the area back and forth.

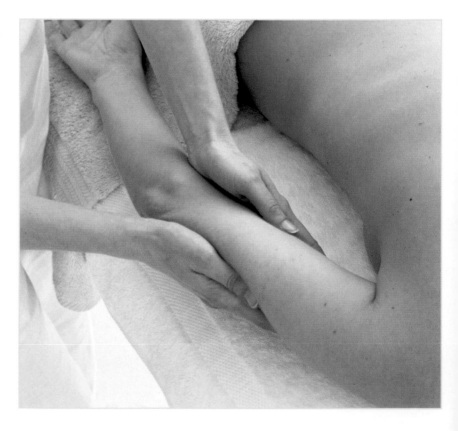

Passive stretching and joint mobilization

In passive stretching the muscle is extended to its natural resting length and held in position for a few seconds before returning it to its shortest resting length. This technique, and joint mobilization, in which the joint is literally moved through its natural range of motion, played a major role in the Swedish system devised by Per Henrik Ling. They encourage the restoration of healthy tissue and pain-free movement. Stretching and mobilization are used together during a massage treatment, but stretching should be practised with caution and only after the body has been warmed up. The movements should be smooth and gentle, avoiding overextending. Make sure that the client is aware of what you are going to do so that they relax instead of resisting the stretch. Ask them to inhale at the start of the stretch or mobilization, exhaling during the movement.

1 To expand the ribcage and stretch the respiratory and arm muscles, slowly slide your hands down your client's arms until you reach the wrist.

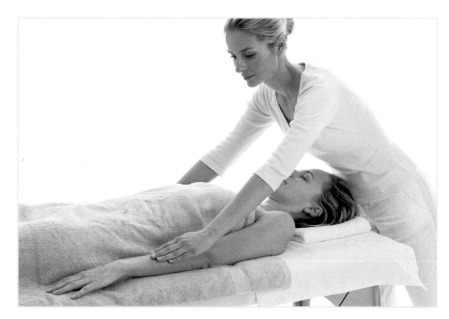

2 Take hold and slowly lift the arms up towards you until comfortably extended, then hold the position for 5–10 seconds before releasing gently. Repeat this stretch two or three times.

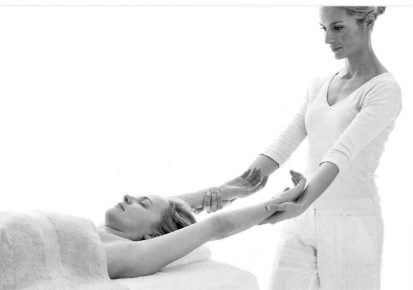

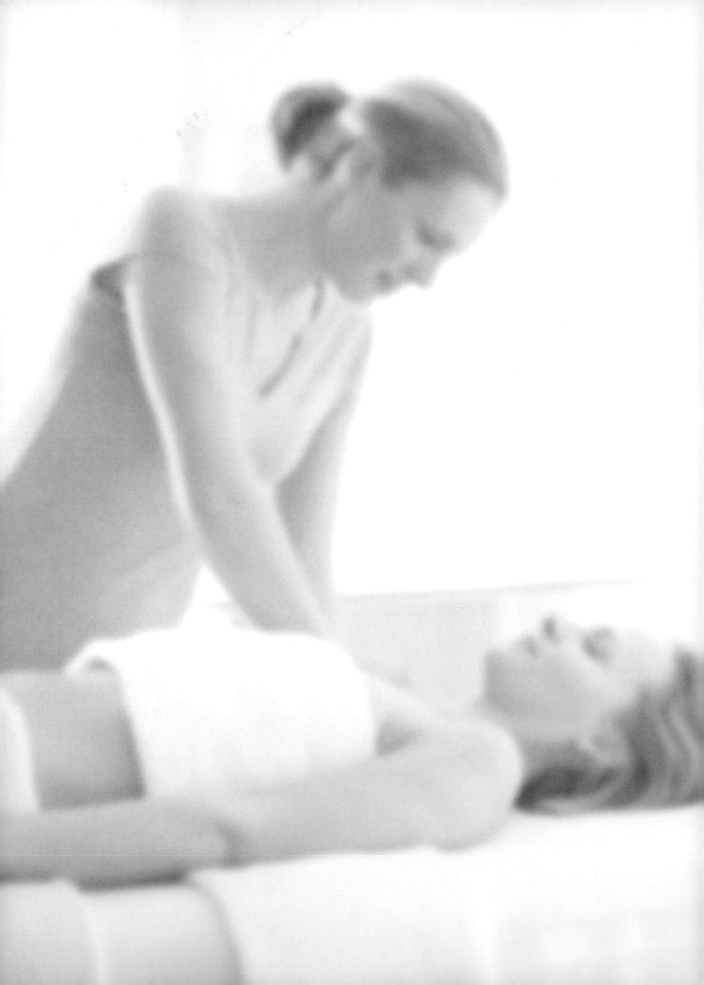

The basic massage sequence

Classical Swedish massage advocates the use of effleurage and petrissage alternately. There is no need to adhere to this routine slavishly though; each treatment will depend on the requirements of the client, and as a massage therapist you will soon develop your own basic routine and build on that. The time spent on each area and the pressure used will also be tailored to achieve the best outcome. Whatever routine is employed, at least one of your hands should maintain contact at all times until the end of the treatment.

Order of practice

The basic massage routine known as the Swedish sequence is easy to understand and memorize and the one most commonly used. The back is often the area requiring the most work and focus and so this is the natural place to begin.

When choosing a section to massage, always apply the basic rule of working towards the heart, applying pressure on the upward stroke, lighter on the return and lifting off pressure over joints. Remember to work either side of the spine and not over it.

The most usual sequence is as follows: With the patient in prone position, start working on the upper back, then move on to the lower back and buttocks, finally work on the back of the legs. Turn the client over (see page 139) and work on the chest and neck, then the face and head. Move on to the arms and hands, then the abdomen, before finishing with the front of the legs and feet.

In some circumstances you may prefer to use an alternative sequence. For example, to build up confidence, particularly with a new client, you may decide to start slowly from the legs upwards, or to relax a very nervous or tense client you could start with the face. If it is a different routine from what they are used to, explain what you are going to do and why, so

Sequence of massage Start your massage with the client in prone position, ensuring they are well supported and the face cradle, if used, is in the correct position.

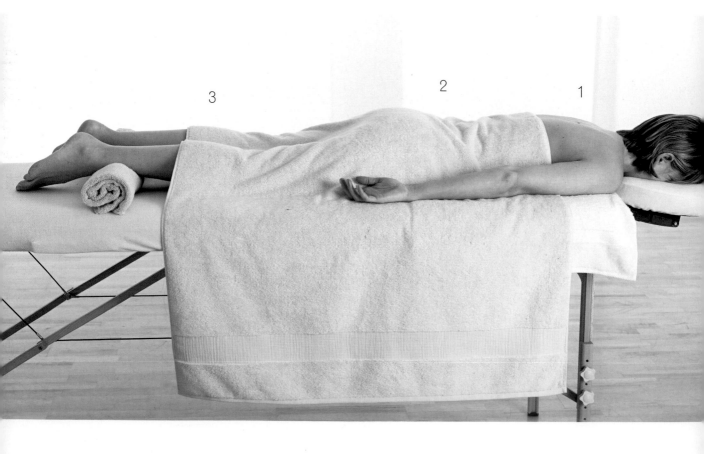

3   2   1

they feel comfortable and tell them whether you would like them to lie prone or supine on the table to start the massage.

A example of an alternative sequence is as follows: Start with the patient in prone position to work on the backs of legs, then move up to the buttocks and lower back, then the upper back, shoulder and neck. Turn the client over to work on the face, then the front of the neck and chest, then arms and hands, the abdomen and finish with the front of the legs and feet.

Another sequence you might find useful starts with the face. This may help a nervous client to relax. Start with the client in a supine position and begin with the face. Then move to the front of the legs before progressing to the abdomen, then front of neck and chest and finally arms and hands. Turn the client over to work on the back, then the upper back, shoulders and neck, before doing the backs of the legs, finishing with the feet.

Supine When turning the client to the supine position for the second half of the massage, remove the face cradle and ensure they are well supported.

SEQUENCE OF MASSAGE

Follow this basic sequence, illustrated below.

Prone:
Contact strokes
1   Upper back
2   Lower back and buttocks
3   Back of legs

Supine:
4   Chest and neck
5   Face and head
6   Arms and hands
7   Abdomen
8   Front of legs
9   Feet
Finishing strokes

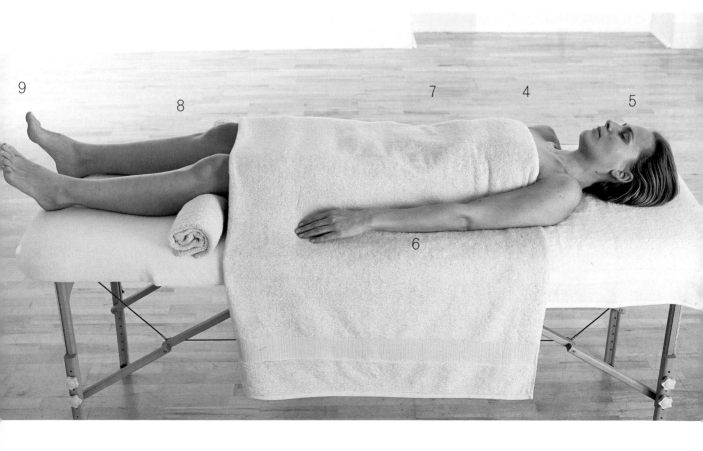

Towels, positioning your client and draping

Massage gives you a licence to touch your clients, but it is important to maintain their modesty and warmth. Only expose those parts of the body that you are actually working on.

Start by using a towels or drapes (bottom sheet, top sheet, one large towel and a smaller towel) with bolsters and pillow for comfort. Warmth is important and if the client is particularly cold an extra blanket can be used or a heated pad under the couch cover. If the client becomes too warm and asks for the drapes to be reduced, always ensure that the breasts, gluteal cleft and genital areas remain covered. The drapes also represent the professional boundaries to operate within.

When moving the drapes during a massage treatment make sure this is done in a simple, unruffled movement. Similarly, when the client is required to turn over, the therapist should hold and anchor the drapes to maintain modesty. To reveal an area, fold the drape back or under

and if it does not remain in place of its own accord, tuck it lightly underneath the body to hold.

Towels are the most commonly used drapes, though some therapists like to use sheets. Both systems require the massage table itself to be covered with a specialized couch cover and, if preferred, disposable paper couch roll on top to avoid seepage of oils.

One large towel is used to drape a male client and two for a female. Make sure the feet are covered to stop the

T formation For female clients, the use of a smaller drape in a T formation to cover the upper torso will give greater flexibility when exposing the abdominal area for massage.

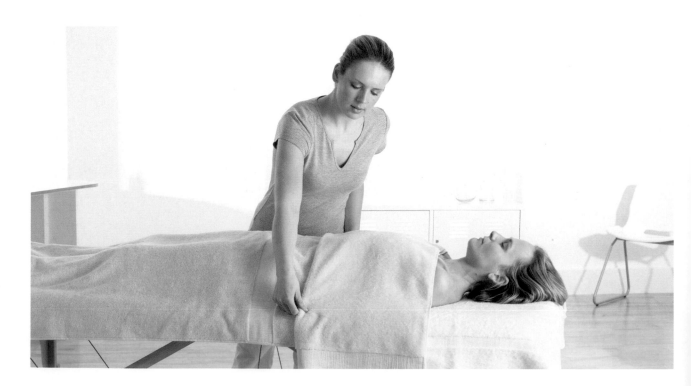

extremities getting cold, using an extra towel if necessary. Ask the client to lie on the table covered in a towel, once they have undressed, before commencing the massage, gently pull the opposite two corners to make sure the body is totally draped. For a female client, place a smaller towel parallel to the top edge of the towel in a T formation over the chest and shoulder areas.

When massaging the abdomen on a female client, the bottom edge of the top towel is fan folded to make a 'bikini top' and the larger towel folded down, exposing the abdomen, ready for massage. The reverse movement will cover the area at the end of the sequence.

When turning from prone to supine, the client should roll towards the therapist. If using a face cradle, ask the client to first move down so that their head is supported on the massage table. Then reach across and take the furthermost corners of the towel in each corresponding hand and, anchoring the nearside edge of the towel by

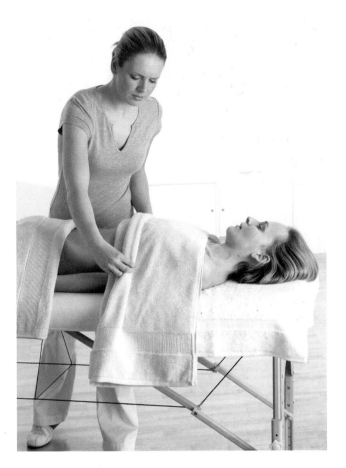

Draping (right) Folding back the smaller drape to the upper edge of the ribcage will allow massage of the abdominal area, maintaining modesty for female clients.

Turning a client (below) When turning from a prone to supine position, ask the client to turn towards the drape you are holding and this will maintain complete modesty.

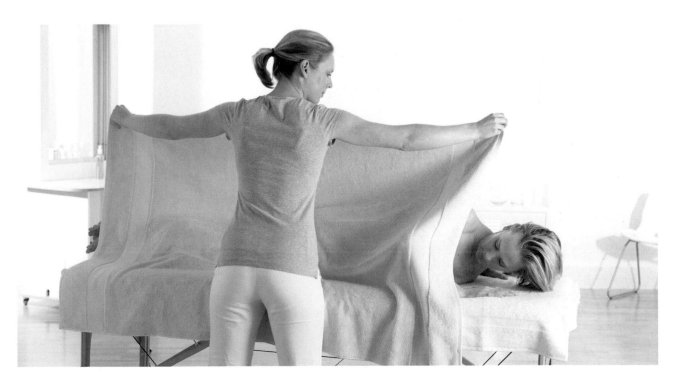

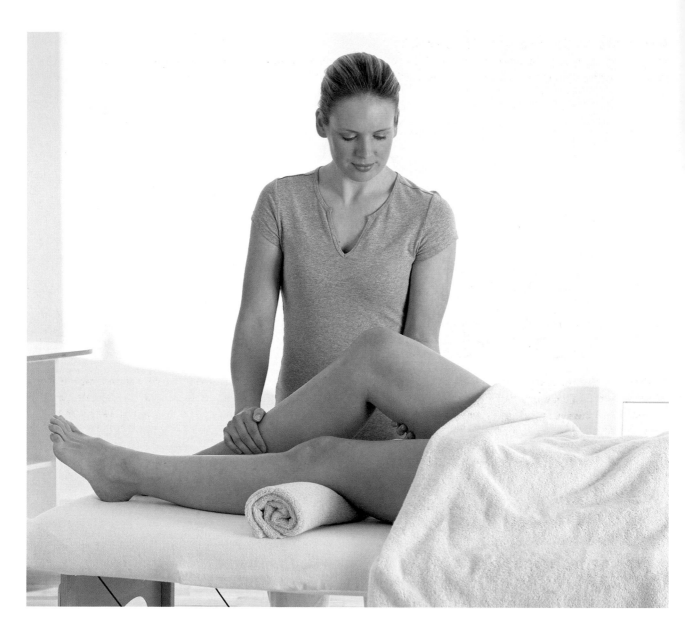

leaning against it, ask the client to face towards you and roll over until supine.

The towel can then be laid back down and bolsters placed under the neck and knees. If starting with the client supine, the same procedure is used to turn them prone. Once in position, ask them to move upwards and place their face comfortably in the face cradle if used. Bolsters should then be put in position under the ankles. Women with large breasts will sometimes find a pillow under the abdomen makes for a more comfortable massage.

Sometimes a client will have a condition that requires them to receive massage lying on their side. In this case the same draping methods are used, but you will also

Bolsters The general rule for bolster support is to place it under the knees when the client is supine and under the ankles when lying prone.

need a selection of pillows to prop up the chest, abdomen and legs. When massaging the back, uncover the area by folding the towel in half lengthways and draping it over the side of the client to secure. The arms and legs should be worked on from the front, with the client draped from the chest downwards. To turn the client the sequence is the same as a prone to supine move, although the pillows will need to be replaced under the drape, which may take some practice to become a smooth operation.

Assisting a client to get off the table

When a client requires assistance to get on and off the table, there are a variety of methods that can be used to enable the drapes to remain in place. The easiest method to help the client off the table is described below:

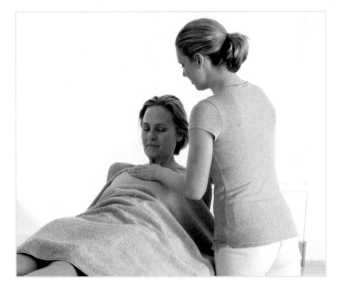

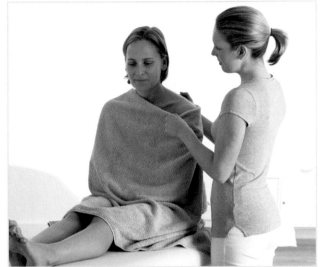

1 Face your client, standing with your hip or thigh leaning against the massage table at their waist level. Place your nearside arm under your client's nearside arm and hold confidently under and slightly behind the shoulder. Slide your arm under the back until supporting both shoulders and grasp the edge of the towel at the same time.

2 Ask your client to move to a sitting position, assisting them with weight transference from your legs, not your back. Pull the drape around their neck and shoulders and secure.

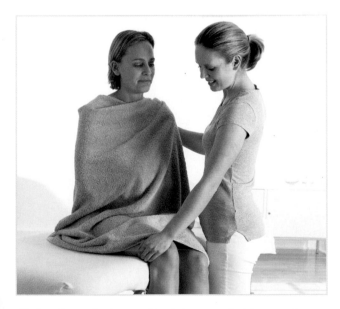

3 Reach over both your client's knees and with cupped hands pull them towards you until their feet dangle off the edge of the table. Maintain the position of the drape and assist further until the client is standing.

If using sheets instead of towels, you will require one large sheet to drape the client. A flat, single-size sheet is the most suitable. As you undrape specific areas, tuck the ends under the client's body to secure. With sheets you are able to cocoon the body and feet, which often gives a feeling of security and nurturing to the client.

Whichever type of drape you choose, draping is an art in itself and a challenge for the new therapist. Be patient and if you accidentally expose a client, acknowledge the fact. If you feel it is necessary, offer a short apology and reposition the drape whilst looking away. A small slip of a drape will not need this attention, simply redress the situation and carry on without any interruption.

The massage sequence

The following pages are a step-by-step guide to the most usual sequence used to apply Swedish massage techniques.

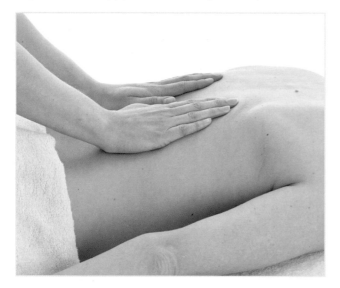

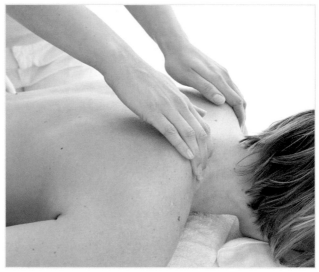

1 Begin with effleurage. Make contact by placing both hands either side of the spine on the sacrum. Glide upwards towards the shoulders, across and around, returning down the sides of the torso with pressure on the upward stroke. To apply more pressure lean your body into your hands. Repeat three to five times.

2 Glide your hands up the back as before, extend the hands over each shoulder, hooking the flats of the fingers into the front shoulder muscles. Pull back towards you and hold before releasing. Return down the sides of the torso.

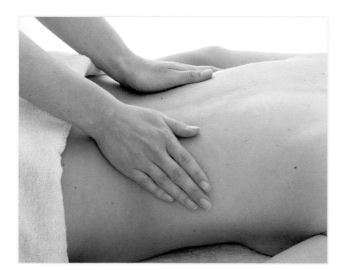

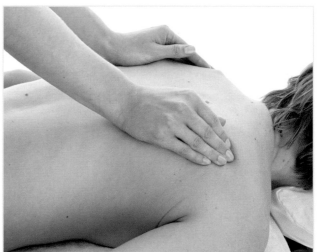

3 Starting at the lower back, push both hands simultaneously out to the sides of the torso, circling back around to meet each other. Continue the stroke, working up the back in sets of circles to the tops of the shoulders and return down the sides of the torso as before. Repeat three to five times.

4 With your hands placed with fingers facing away from each other apply petrissage by leaning the heels of the hands into the groove either side of the spine, manipulating the soft tissue between the heel of the hands and the fingers and return. Work up the length of the back to the scapula, decreasing pressure over the kidney area.

Working the shoulder from the side

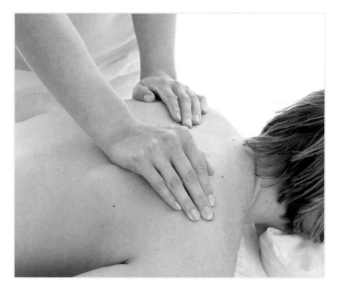

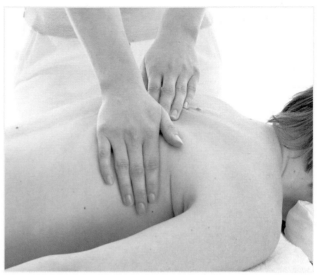

1 Working side-on to your client, one hand maintaining contact, apply one-handed petrissage on the side furthest away from you up towards the scapula, before moving to the other side and repeating.

2 Check the position of your client's arm. You may wish to gently move it away from the torso to enable easier access to the area you are going to massage. Still in a side-on position, knead the area below the armpit on the far side by pushing the web of the hand into the muscle, pick up and squeeze the soft tissue between the fingers and thumb before releasing. As you release with one hand, pick up with the other, working them towards each other.

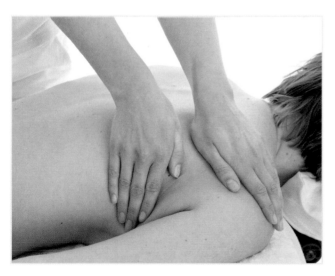

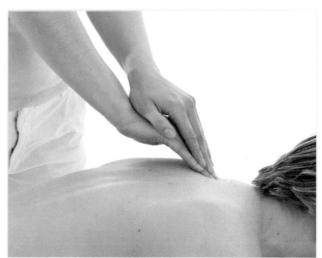

3 Working the same area, place the flats of the hands on the top of the scapula and effleurage downwards towards the top of the arm, circling back to repeat. When returning add a slight lift and pull in order to open up the area.

4 Returning to the original position and working on the nearest side, apply circling strokes by placing one hand on top of the other, fingers straight and relaxed. With the finger pads, slowly rotate over the soft tissue either side of the spine, working upwards towards the shoulders. Work from the base of the neck outwards along the shoulder line.

Working the shoulder from the side *continued*

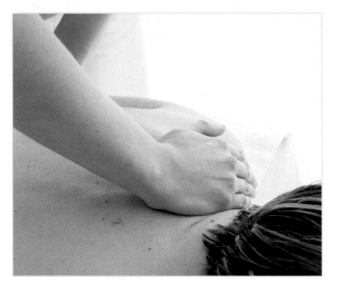

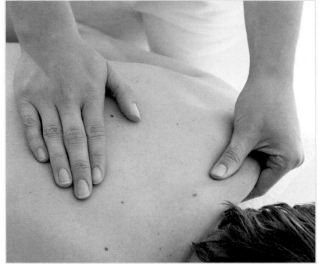

5 Placing the heel of one hand over the shoulder muscle, maintaining contact with the other, hook the flats of the fingers into the muscle at the front of the shoulder as before, then push the heel into the soft tissue until the hand glides off the shoulder. Repeat three to five times.

6 In the same position, pick up the muscle between the thumb and fingers of one hand, applying pressure, squeeze firmly, moving along the length of the muscle inwards towards the base of the neck. As you release, effleurage over the area with the other hand in the opposite direction, outwards to the edge of the shoulder. Repeat this squeeze and soothe stroke three to five times before moving to the other side to repeat the last two movements on the other shoulder.

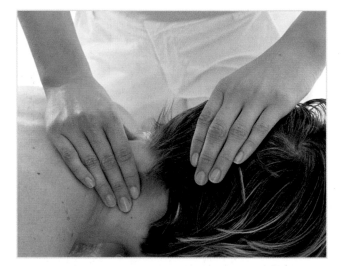

7 With the web of one hand placed over the base of the neck, using the thumb and finger pads, work up towards the base of the skull in a scoop and squeeze action, taking care not to pinch the skin or work too far forward towards the throat. A more dynamic variation is to work with both hands, one travelling upwards whilst the other travels downwards, lifting off one following the other.

Working the back and shoulder from the head

At this stage the back area can often be finished off with light effleurage and stroking. If further work is required, keeping contact, position yourself at the head of the table in order to apply a reverse effleurage sequence. Reverse effleurage of the back is a wonderful flowing sequence with varying pressures following an hourglass shape over the contours of the client's body.

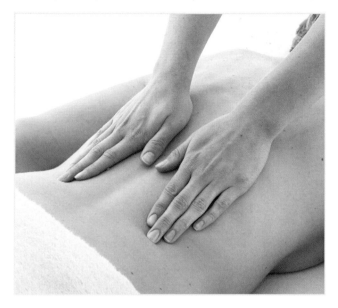

1 Place both hands either side of the spine at the top of the scapulas and, applying pressure, glide down the length of the back.

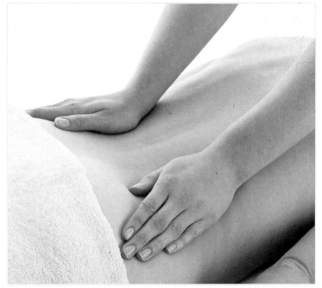

2 At the top of the buttocks (gluteals) turn the hands outwards and return up the sides of the torso, using light pressure and a very slight pulling action.

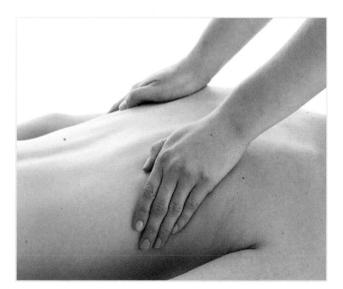

3 As you reach the base of the scapula, turn your hands inwards, wrists and elbows facing out and following the contours of the torso, increase the pressure and effleurage outward towards the tops of the arms and over the deltoid muscles.

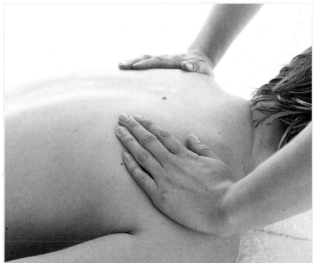

4 As your hands cup the tops of the arms, rotate them so that the flats of the fingers slide under the shoulders, the heel of hands acting as stabilizers and glide up to the base of the neck, applying deeper pressure.

Working the back and shoulder from the head *continued*

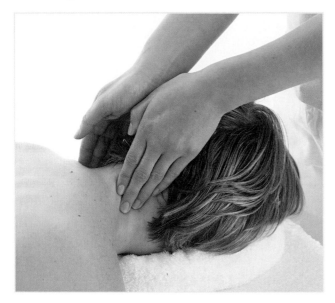

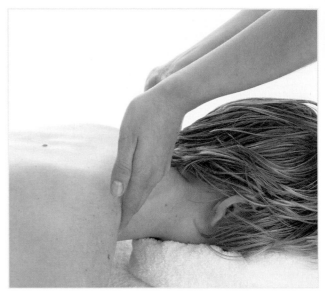

5 From the base of the neck, glide up either side of the spine, meeting at the base of the skull.

6 You can then either lift off to finish or repeat the stroke, keeping contact and gliding your hands back down the neck to the starting point at the top of the scapula.

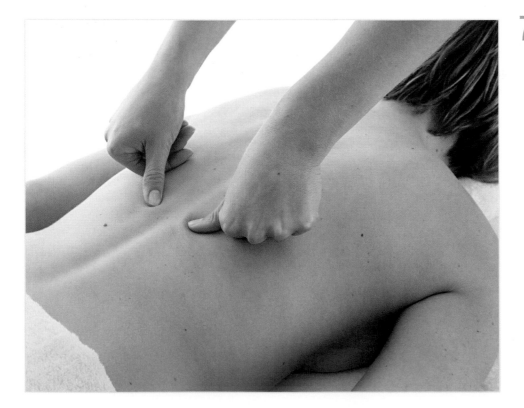

7 You may also wish to integrate some friction or tapotement strokes into the back sequence where appropriate, particularly over areas of deep tension or where stimulation is required.

Working the spine

Much tension is held around the spine and a combination of effleurage and deep friction can be very effective in relaxing the muscles that 'guard' this important part of the anatomy.

Always avoid pressure directly on the vertebrae and work either side of the spine.

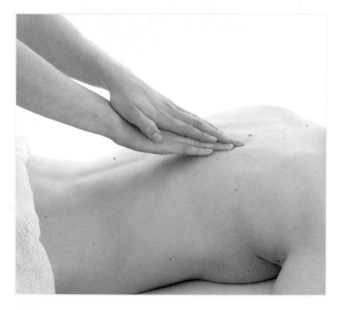

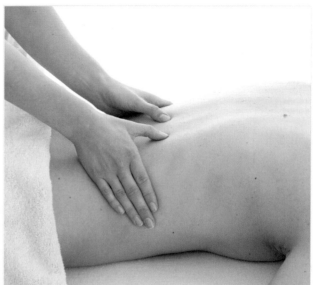

1 Make contact at the base of the spine, using reinforced effleurage. With one hand on top of the other, glide up one side of the spine applying medium pressure. On reaching the top of the shoulder, lift off the pressure, glide across and down the opposite side of the spine. You are then in a position to reverse the sequence with pressure on the upward stroke. This allows the muscle on both sides of the spine to be worked in the same way without losing contact.

2 Once you have warmed up the area with effleurage, working from the same starting point as before, place hands either side of the spine, thumbs apart in order to apply the friction stroke of circling along the muscle. The pads of the thumbs move in small circular movements, whilst at the same time applying deep pressure and moving up the length of the muscle before sweeping gently back down to the start.

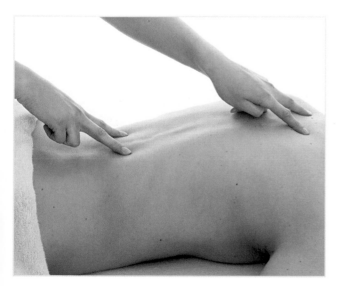

3 Finish this sequence along the spine with the raking stroke. Applied with the index and middle finger of the hand forming a 'V' shape, the fingertips are placed either side of the spine and pulled down a section of the muscles, one hand after the other until the whole area is worked. Raking is a great connecting stroke and finishing with it will allow you to move your position around the table or work on another section of the body without losing contact.

Working the lower back and buttocks

This sequence should only be used if the client is happy to have the area worked as it is one of the least exposed parts of the body and therefore your touch needs to be confident and reassuring. The gluteal muscles that make up most of the buttocks are large muscles that can store much tension and a massage excluding them may feel incomplete.

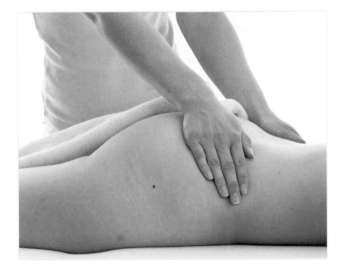

1 With the client in prone position, position yourself on one side at thigh level in order to massage the opposite side. Make contact on the sacrum with the flats of your hands and circle broadly over the lower back area, using hands alternately. This will result in the pelvis rocking from side to side, relaxing and releasing tension whilst warming the area.

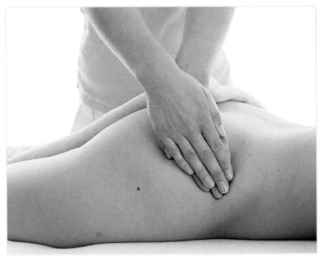

2 Using double-handed effleurage, glide up the side of the lower back furthest away from you, pushing up over the top and side of the buttock before returning to the start position. The pressure should be on the upward stroke and as you draw the hands around the sides of the buttock. Repeat two or three times.

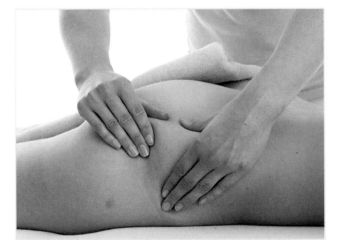

3 Moving sideways on to the table, facing opposite the buttock you are working on, knead deeply the muscle by scooping up the soft tissue between the fingers and thumbs. Squeezing and wringing, work around the entire buttock using a flowing rhythm and alternating pressure and speed when required.

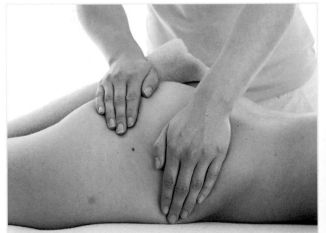

4 With slightly cupped hands, use the flats of the fingers to pull upwards from the hip to the top of the buttock, one hand following the other.

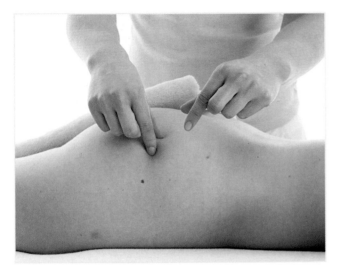

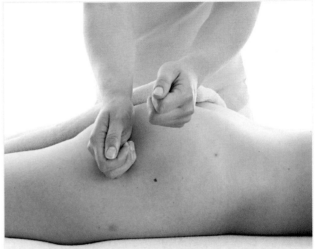

5 Still using hands alternately, apply tapotement to stimulate circulation in the area. Pinching or pounding are the strokes used on the posterior thigh and gluteal regions. Grasp small pockets of soft tissue between the thumb and finger pads and lift slightly before releasing in a rapid, consistent movement.

6 With your knuckles facing downwards, pound in a light knocking action. Start gently, allowing your hands to bounce off the buttock at an even pace.

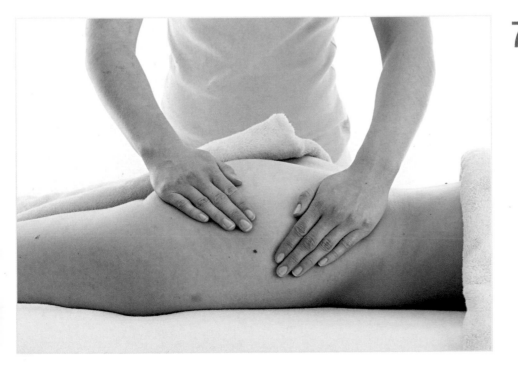

7 Finally, calm the area with a couple of long effleurage strokes. At the end of the sequence move to the other side and repeat.

Working the backs of the legs

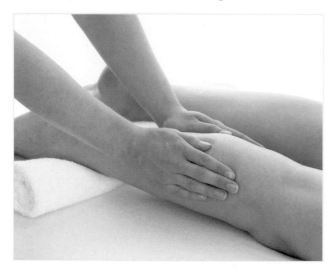

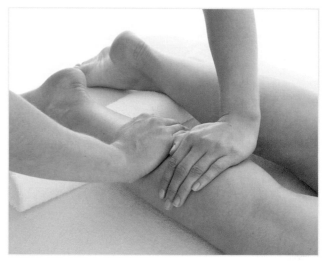

1 With the client lying prone, position yourself in line with the ankles at the side you are starting with. Apply flat-handed effleurage, gliding from the ankles up the length of the limb, lifting off the pressure as you pass over the back of the knee. On reaching the thigh area, push the outside hand over the gluteal and around the hip, whilst extending the other hand to a level that is not invasive on the inner thigh. Synchronize both hands to return down the sides of the legs, finish on the tops of the ankles with a slight pull.

2 Turn your hands inwards, wrists and elbows out and repeat the stroke using cupped effleurage, the left hand working in front of the right. When you reach the thigh, rotate the outside hand over the gluteal muscle and hip whilst the other hand moves around to the inner thigh, maintaining modesty as before. Glide down the leg, cupping the sides between the thumb and fingers of each hand until pulling off at the ankle.

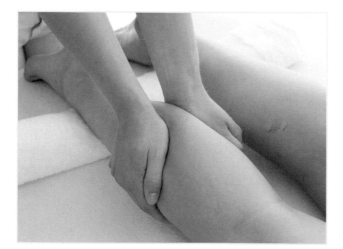

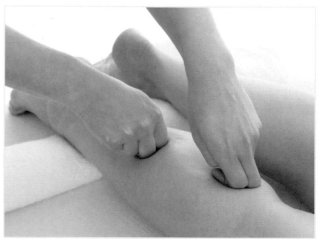

3 Keeping both hands at the base of the calf, apply double-handed petrissage. With the heels of hands alongside each other, lean into the soft tissue, pushing outwards whilst lifting and squeezing. Work the length of the calf muscle. To work the area above the knee, keep contact with one hand and, using the outside hand, apply petrissage over the thigh and gluteal muscles.

4 At this stage you can also apply a knuckling stroke by making your hands into relaxed fists and, one after the other, run the knuckles upwards over the muscles, one hand making contact as the other lifts off. This stroke allows you to apply varying pressures and speeds over the back and sides of the upper leg and buttock.

Leg drainage

The muscles of the backs of the legs are long and often hold concentrated areas of tension and a build-up of lactic acid.

Drainage strokes will assist with circulation and help break down any adhesions and storage of toxins.

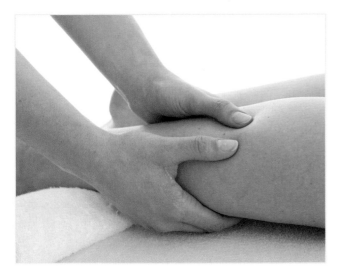

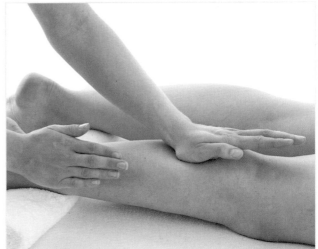

1 Starting below the calf, place the pads of the thumbs on the backs of the legs with the rest of the hand in a supporting position and using alternate thumbs press against the soft tissue, working up the calf and thigh avoiding the back of the knee. Each stroke should be short and firm and applied in a regular rhythm.

2 Glide your hands back to the start point and this time, instead of applying the stroke with the thumb pads, use the heels of the hands, pushing them into the soft tissue using alternate, deep, broad strokes. As with the thumb stroke, the movement should be short, firm and applied in a regular rhythm, working slowly up the length of the leg.

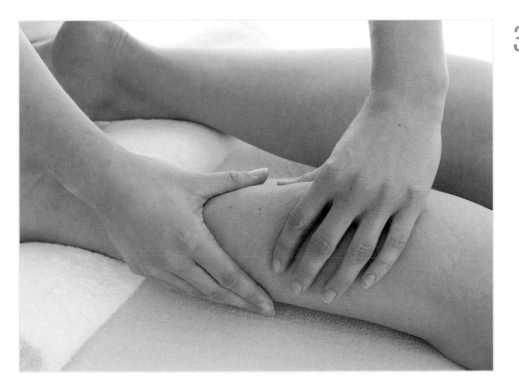

3 To finish, you can apply a few long strokes of flat-handed effleurage or work back down the leg with petrissage strokes before finishing with light effleurage. The backs of the legs, thighs and buttocks are particularly soft and fleshy, so are ideal to integrate kneading, wringing and rolling strokes into the massage. If the area is sensitive or painful it could be the result of lower back or sciatic problems and massage may also bring referred release of tension in these areas.

Leg lift

To work the ankles and feet or relax the calf muscles, it is easier to work with the leg bent at the knee. This position is often used when applying advanced massage such as sports and remedial massage because the muscle is more relaxed and easier to manipulate. The therapist should lean into the massage table and allow the top of the client's foot and ankle to rest on their nearside shoulder for support. This leaves both hands free to manipulate the leg from the ankle upwards.

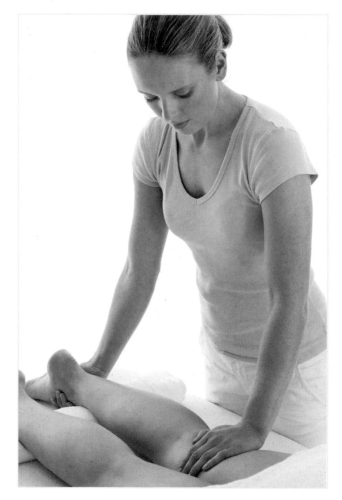

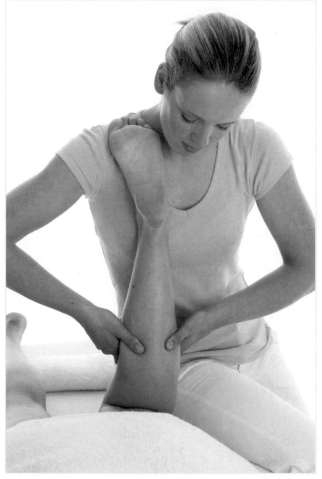

1 Position yourself at the side of the leg you wish to work on and place one hand under the ankle and the other on the back of the knee.

2 Very slowly lift the lower leg until it is perpendicular to the table. You can tell whether your client is relaxed or not by noting whether they 'help' you raise the leg or surrender to your touch.

Working the ankle

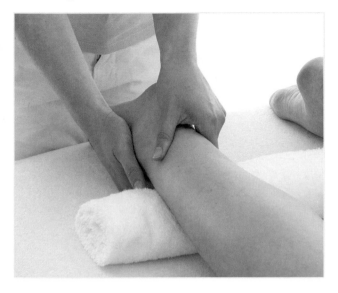

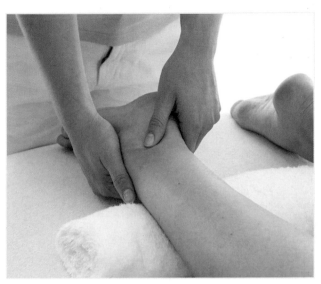

1 Supporting the ankle with one hand, use the pads of your thumb and fingers of the other to scoop and squeeze the Achilles tendon around the ankle. This tendon is often very tight and prone to injury. Massage can warm and relax the area, and is often part of sports-injury prevention and maintenance programmes. It helps to restore flexibility and reduces any oedema present.

2 Continue to work with the pads of the thumbs and fingers, applying circular friction around the ankle bone, working one side of the leg and then the other.

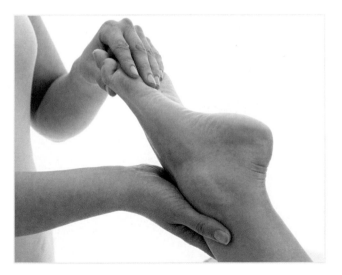

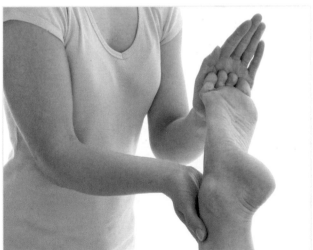

3 Finish off the work on the ankles with some passive stretching and joint mobilizations. Support the leg just above the ankle with one hand; with the other hand, grasp the foot around the top and ball in a confident, firm hold. Slowly rotate the foot in wide circles, clockwise and then anti-clockwise, to the full range of its flexibility.

4 With the ankle supported in one hand, use the other to push down the toes and balls of the foot until it reaches the point of resistance and hold. From this point pull the front of the foot backwards, at the same time applying pressure to the heel with the supporting hand. The aim of this movement is to flex the ankle, at the same time stretching the foot and front of the leg.

Working the foot

The foot can be worked either in the leg bent position or with the client supine on the massage table, the ankle supported by a small bolster or rolled up towel. This will depend on where in your routine you decide to massage the feet. With a bent leg it can be added at the end of the back of legs routine before repositioning the leg back on the table, ready for the client to turn over. The strokes are applied with one hand, the other supporting the foot. Alternatively it can be the closure routine following the front of the legs, with the client resting on the massage table. In this case both hands can be used to apply the strokes.

You may wish to concentrate on the feet when there is not enough time to complete a full body massage as they affect the whole of the body. The feet are immensely complex structures containing 26 small bones. They carry the full body weight and contain thousands of nerve endings and reflexes that connect to the rest of the body.

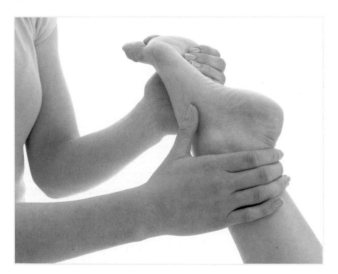

1 Supporting the sole of the foot with one hand, use the pads of the thumb of the other to apply circle friction slowly and deeply over the top of the foot. Once the whole foot has been worked, apply pressure in small short strokes, working along the grooves between the tendons in a direction from the ankle to the toes.

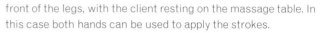
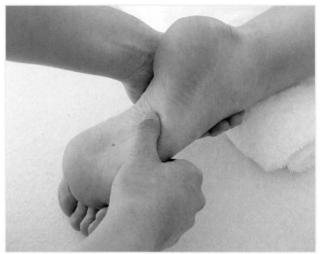

2 With one hand supporting the ankle, place the other around the top of the foot with the thumb resting on the sole. Using the pad of the thumb, work across the whole of the sole, applying circular friction strokes, starting at the heel and ending at the ball. Make sure you pressure is firm and confident as light strokes may tickle or feel annoying.

3 You can also add some cross-fibre strokes, working over the ball of the foot, extending out to the edges of the foot if there is built up tension apparent.

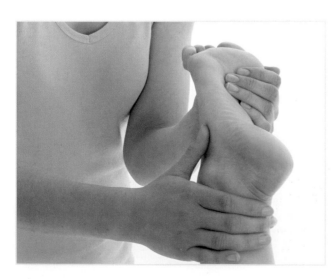

Working the shoulders, neck and scalp

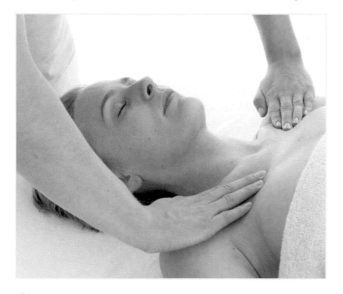

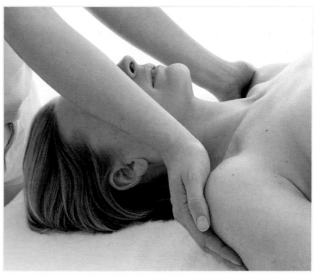

1 Make contact on the upper chest just below the collarbone with the flats of both hands, fingers facing towards each other. Making sure you do not lean into the chest, slowly effleurage by drawing the hands away from each other towards the shoulders, applying firm but not heavy pressure.

2 As your hands reach the top of the shoulders, bring the heels of the hands inwards, so that the fingers scoop underneath, working up the back of the neck until your fingers meet.

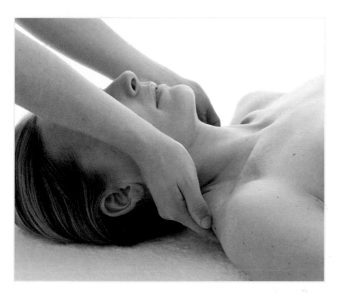

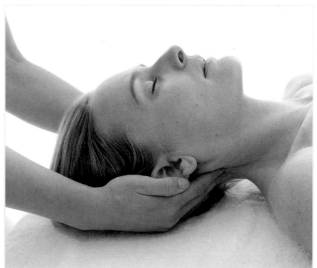

3 Continue up the back of the neck to the base of the skull and release, repeating three to five times.

4 On the last stroke, if the client is happy for you to do so, follow through the back of the head, releasing at the crown, in a continuous slow gliding movement. Do not be tempted to lift the head. If this is the end of a massage sequence, a relaxing way to finish is to follow the scalp routine (see page 159).

Neck stretches

Whilst working the shoulders, neck and scalp, you are in a position to integrate some simple stretches as extensions of the long strokes. Some clients will feel relaxed and their heads will feel 'heavy' in your hands, others may resist slightly at first, so simply carry on with the next stroke. These stretches will help to release tension held in the neck and shoulders.

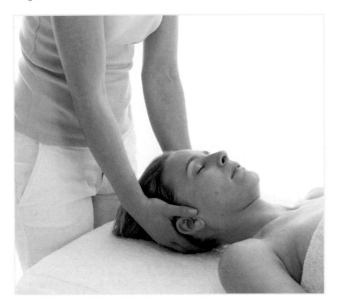

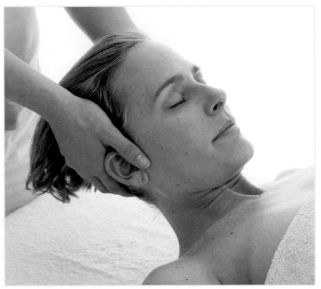

1 At the point your hands meet behind the back of the neck in the last sequence, cup your hands one on top of the other, with thumbs tucked in, and gently pull your hands towards you, at the same time leaning back a little. This will exert a gentle stretch on the neck and tops of shoulders before you release the cupped hands and continue up the back of the neck and scalp.

2 Once you have completed the stroke and released at the crown, using slightly cupped hands, position them firmly under the head with your fingers resting on the base of the skull. Lift the head upwards, bringing the chin towards the chest. Ask the client to breathe in at the start of the lift and out when at chest level.

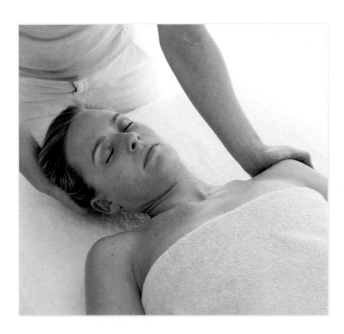

3 As you bring the head back down, move one of your supporting hands under the nape of the neck and lift slightly, allowing the head to tilt backwards. Straighten back to the level or resting position without extending the neck backwards and, supporting the head with both hands, carefully place back on the massage couch. Keeping one support hand in place at the back of the skull, move the head very slowly in the direction of one shoulder, at the same time placing your other hand on the opposite shoulder, applying medium pressure. Hold the position for a few seconds before releasing and returning to the centre, supporting with both hands. Repeat on the other side by reversing your hands. This movement stretches right along the top of the shoulder and the side of the neck, where tension often builds up.

Working the shoulders front and back

Once the area has been warmed up with effleurage, make your hands into fists and make contact on the upper chest below the collarbone as before.

Work over the front of the chest and around the fleshier areas in front of the armpits, by circling the knuckles and rotating the hands, simultaneously applying the friction stroke of knuckling. The stroke can also be extended over the upper arms and applied with one hand whilst keeping contact with the other. If the chest area is hairy, be careful not to pull at the hairs as this could cause discomfort.

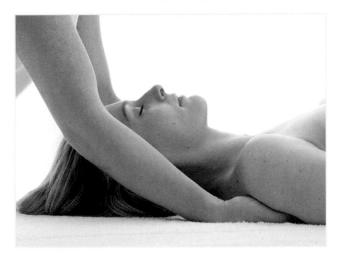

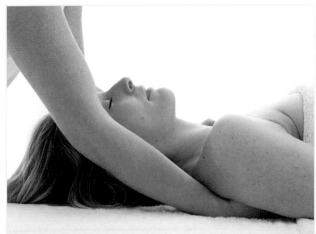

1 Place your hands, fingers together, on the upper chest just below the collarbone. Glide them away from each other and as your hands reach the top of the shoulders, bring the heel of hands inwards, so that the fingers scoop underneath the shoulder. Push down the soft tissue along the outer edge of the scapula, reaching as far as possible towards the waist without overstretching yourself.

2 Curve your fingers very slightly and pull back upwards, tracing the natural groove diagonally across the back.

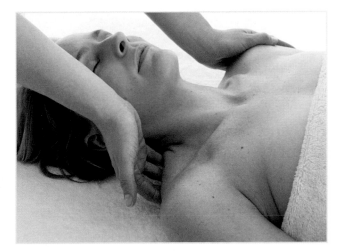

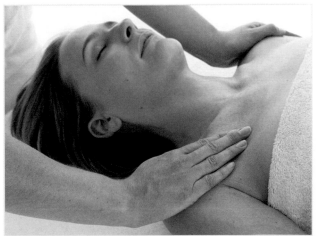

3 Follow the lower edge of the scapula to the neck and the base of the skull. Making small circles with the pads of your fingers, work along the edge of the base of the skull outwards from the centre before returning to repeat the whole sequence.

4 Once again, place your hands, fingers together on the upper chest just below the collarbone, glide them away from each other, and as your hands reach the top of the shoulders, bring the heel of hands inwards, circling the shoulder joint.

Working the shoulders front and back *continued*

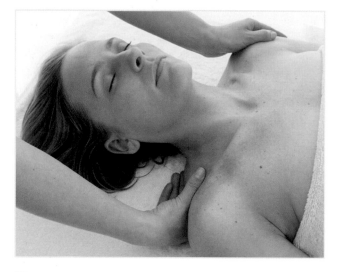

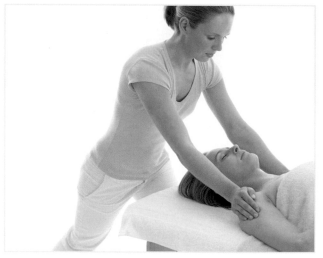

5 Using your thumb placed over the front of the shoulder, supported by the fingers behind, grasp the soft tissue between them and, leaning into the muscle, squeeze along the length, up the back of the neck to the base of the skull.

6 To finish off work on the shoulders, place the heel of both hands on the tops of the shoulders, lightly resting the fingers on the fronts. Lean inwards, applying pressure horizontally in a direction towards the client's feet, hold and release. You may find it useful to breathe in on contact and release, and outwards when applying pressure. If a client is very tense you could start the treatment of this area with the same movement, additionally pushing one shoulder and then the other in a relaxing rhythm to establish trust and loosen the area.

Spinal stretch

For this stroke you will need the participation of your client as it is not a totally passive stretch.

It may take a little practice before you can smoothly integrate the spinal stretch into your massage sessions and it should not be attempted if the client is much larger or heavier than yourself. The key to this stretch is to ensure that the pull always originates from your pelvis and not the shoulders.

Explain to your client what you are doing and ask them to arch their back a little, enabling you to to push your hands, palms upwards, and forearms as far under the back as possible. Position each arm and hand either side of the spine, resting the top of the shoulder in the crook of your elbow. Once you feel the client relaxing into your arms, using slightly curved fingers, pull your hands up the soft tissue either side of the spine whilst moving your own body backwards. As you travel the length of the spine up to the neck, releasing at the back of the head, the whole area is pleasantly stretched out.

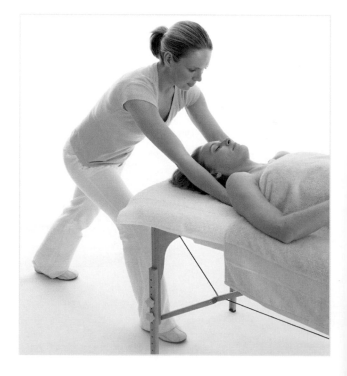

Working the scalp

The scalp, just as other parts of the body, can store tension and stiffness that respond well to massage.

The thin muscle layer covering the skull tightens with tension and stress, causing headaches and anxiety. Massage helps to loosen the muscle and improve circulation, inducing relaxation and improving hair condition. This sequence can be added to the chest and neck or facial routines and can be applied with or without oil.

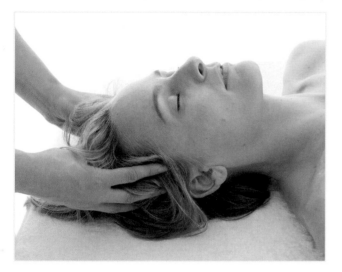

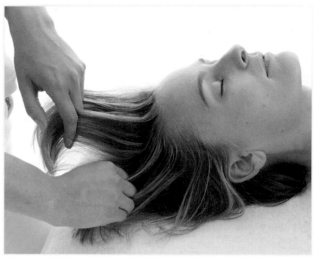

1 Using both hands, make contact either side of the head above the tops of the ears and, using the finger pads, apply pressure, rotating the fingers slowly all over the scalp in a 'shampooing' movement. Gradually increase the pace and make sure the pressure is deep enough to move the scalp. Focus around the ears and above the forehead.

2 With your hands positioned down and palms towards you, draw the fingers slowly through the hair from the scalp outwards in a 'combing' or 'raking' movement along the whole length. Work across the centre of the scalp first and then either side.

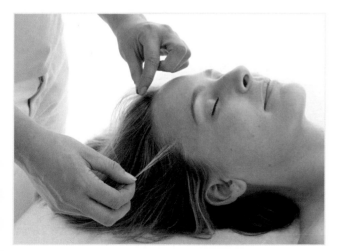

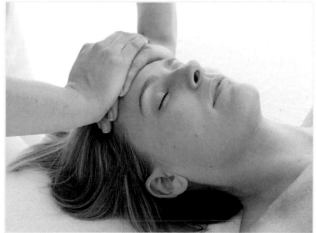

3 Use the thumb and forefinger of one hand to gently take hold of a small tuft of hair at the roots and with a slight pull, slide along the length and off, repeating with the other hand. Work your way along the hairline from the centre outwards in a gentle rhythmical motion.

4 To finish, rest your hands on the forehead, one on top of the other and hold position for around 10–20 seconds before removing very slowly, one at a time. It is important for your working position to be comfortable as any shift of balance or movement, however slight, will feel magnified by the client and may break their relaxation.

Working the face

The face is probably the smallest, most sensitive of the areas that you will apply massage to and so your strokes have to be tailored accordingly. Many movements require only the use of the finger pads and very light pressure, making sure that the skin is not dragged or pulled. The movements will be small so the working position needs to be one where you avoid overtensing your shoulders.

You may also find it useful to synchronize your breathing and movement; breathing in on contact and out on the stroke.

You may not need to use any additional massage medium as your hands will be oiled from the previous sequence. However, the use of a premixed aromatherapy oil such as rose absolute on the temples can enhance the treatment. Before starting, check if your client is wearing contact lenses and if so, omit working over the eyelids from the sequence. Remember also to ask your client for feedback, as sensitivity and comfort levels will vary greatly from person to person.

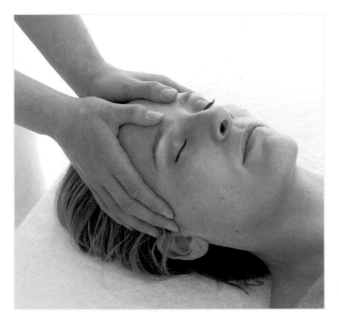

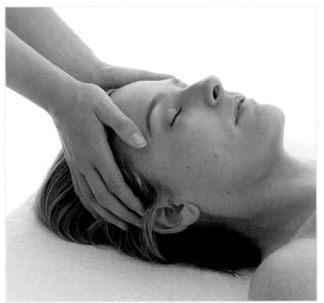

1 Rest your hands on the forehead in a gradual but confident movement, the thumb tips just above the eyebrows and the heels of the hands in the centre of the forehead, adjacent to each other. The web of the hand is extended, with the fingers following the curve of the face. Do not push downwards but maintain a firm pressure for 10–20 seconds.

2 Leaning slightly forward, transfer your weight to the thumbs and slowly glide them across the forehead, outwards towards the ears, keeping them straight and relaxed. As the thumbs make contact with the rest of the hand, lift them off and return to a position slightly above the last. Repeat this way until you have moved up the whole of the forehead to the hairline.

Working the eyes, nose and cheeks

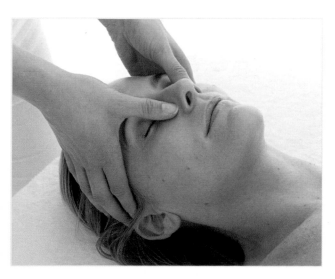

1 Return to the original starting position with the pads of the thumbs placed directly on the inner edge of the eyebrows. Leaning forward, transfer your weight to the thumbs and glide them outwards along the length of the brow to the front of the ears. Lift off the thumbs, keeping the rest of the hand in position and return to repeat the stroke as required.

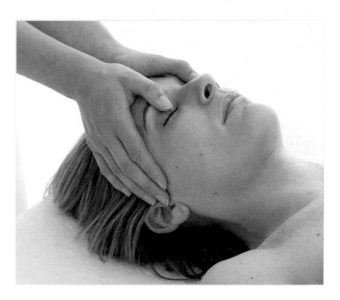

2 If the client is not wearing contact lenses, ask them to close their eyes and, as before using the thumb pads only, smoothly and gently glide over the eyelids from the inner corners, outwards towards the ears. It is important not to apply any pressure or drag the skin over this very delicate area.

3 Returning the thumbs back to a position either side of the top of the nose, use the rest of the hand to support whilst maintaining contact. Glide the pads of the thumbs down the sides of the nose until they reach the nostrils, lift off and return to repeat or keep in position ready for the next part of the sequence. It is important to keep the pressure light to avoid inhibiting breathing.

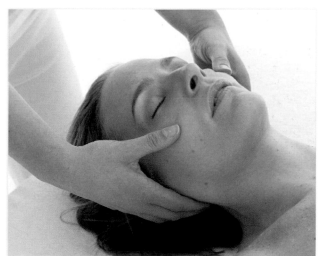

4 With your thumbs in position at the edge of the nostrils, either side of the nose, move the heels of the hands outwards, curving the fingers around the back of the neck for support. Glide the thumbs outwards over the cheeks towards the hairline just above the ears. Lift off and repeat working in strips, ending just below the lower cheekbone.

Working the chin and jawline

The masseters or muscles used for chewing are the only muscles of the face that attach to bone.

The jawbone articulates with the temporomandibular joint, enabling speech and eating, and is often an area of tension.

Some people grind their teeth while sleeping. The location of the muscles can be found by clenching the teeth; this causes the muscles to rise and tense up so that they can be felt through the skin in front of and below the ears.

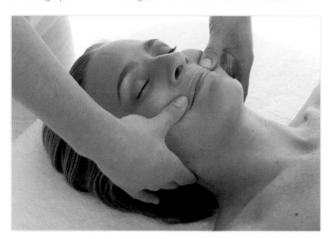

1 Position your hands around your client's face with the flat of the thumbs placed centrally between the nose and the upper lip facing each other, apply medium pressure and slowly glide outwards to the edge of the upper lip. Return and repeat as required. The stroke will want to follow a natural groove, but avoid dragging the skin by working in a straight line rather than downwards towards the lips.

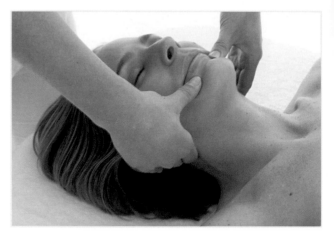

2 With your thumbs positioned as before, place them between the lower lip and the chin. Apply deeper pressure than that on the upper lip, glide outwards to the end of the lower lip, lift off the thumbs, return and repeat as required. You can vary this stroke by lifting the pressure on and off in small strokes, working across the area rather than employing one gliding stroke.

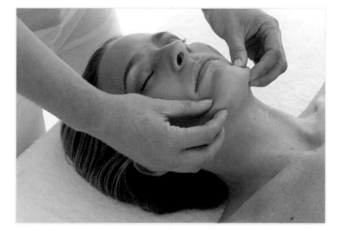

3 Place your thumbs directly below the centre of the lips, curving the fingers underneath the jaw for support. Take the jaw firmly between the finger and thumb pads, pushing into the jaw at the same time. Slowly rotate the thumb pads, keeping the fingers in place and work along the jaw to the ears. A variation on this stroke is to take the jaw firmly between the fingers and thumbs and squeeze along the jaw outwards from the centre to the ears.

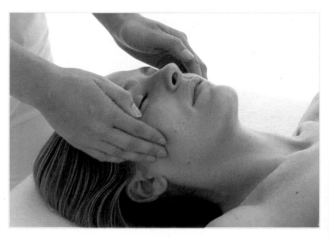

4 Finish off by locating the jaw sockets and with the middle three fingers, lean in slightly and rotate on the spot three or four times in order to relieve any tension. The fingers should be able to naturally locate this position just below the earlobes.

Working the cheeks and ears

In traditional Chinese medicine, points on the ear are believed to correspond to parts of the whole body, just as points on the foot correspond to body parts in the discipline of reflexology. This could be one reason why these strokes are so pleasurable to receive, making this a suitable way to complete your massage treatment.

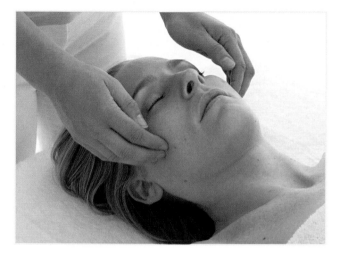

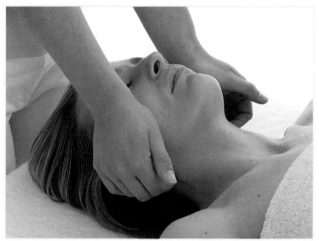

1 Using the pads of the middle fingers make contact centrally on the lower cheekbone and apply pressure, very slowly rotating them in a small circle. Work over the whole of the cheekbone in sections ending at the ears, lifting off just enough to move to the next section without dragging the skin. The pressure should be light unless the massage is to relieve symptoms of a head cold, when pressure the client is comfortable with can be applied.

2 Place the heels of your hands on the top of the cheekbones either side of the nose with fingers pointed towards the ears and slowly glide outwards over the whole cheek area towards the ears.

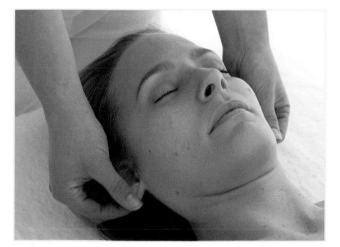

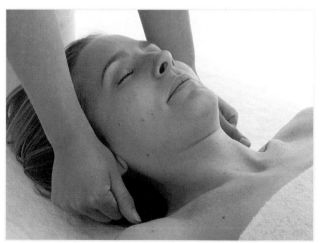

3 With the heels of the hands on top of the ears and the fingers underneath, grasp the ears and very gently stretch them away from the side of the head. Squeeze the earlobes between the thumb and index finger pads and rotate slowly, working up the entire rim of the ear before returning to the lobe.

4 Cup your hands over each ear, with the heels of the hands on top and fingers underneath, then slowly slide your hands downwards and off the ears using a subtle stretching action rather than a pull. Repeat if required.

Working the arms and hands

The muscles and joints of the shoulder are very hard-working and allow the arms and hands to perform manipulative and heavy physical activities. Weight trainers and body builders overdevelop the biceps, triceps and pectorals in order to push their lifting limits. The elbow and flexor muscles of the forearm allow the hands to grip and lift at many levels, whether it is for carrying a bag or participating in sports such as golf, tennis or rowing. The wrist, being a very narrow tunnel filled with tendons, nerves and blood vessels, is constantly at work and so prone to injury, often caused by repetitive strain. Massage plays an important part in maintaining flexibility and releasing tensions that are often experienced in these areas.

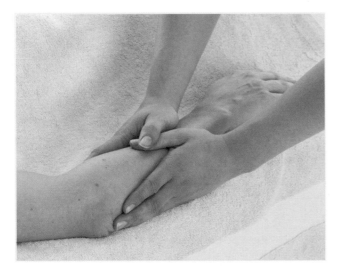

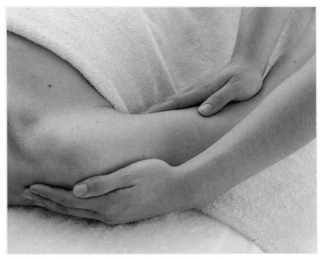

1 Positioning yourself in line with the client's wrist, make contact on the forearm with your hands next to each other. Overlap your thumbs to enable your hands to encase the arm and effleurage slowly up the length of the arm, leaning into the muscle.

2 As you reach the upper arm, separate the hands and glide the outside hand to the top of the shoulder and rotate your wrist, enabling you to effleurage over the shoulder and around the underside of the arm.

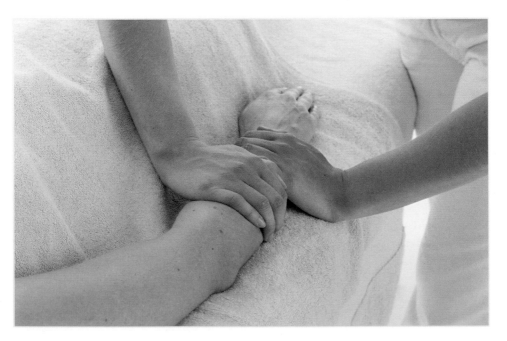

3 With both hands, return down the sides of the arm to just above the wrist, ready to repeat the stroke. You can also apply the stroke with cupped effleurage, which is particularly useful when working on very small or slim arms.

Arm drainage

The next two strokes encourage the circulation of blood and lymph and help relax any tightness or rigidity in the muscles and fascia. The arms are often overworked, which causes this tension and strain. Work the forearm, moving along the upper arm until the whole limb has been massaged. Finish off with two or three long effleurage strokes covering the whole length of the arm from wrist to shoulder.

Stretching

Passive stretching will stretch out the joint and connective tissues of the shoulder, toning and improving range of movement. The stimulation of synovial fluid that 'oils' any joint will also promote ease of movement. Explain to the client what you are going to do so that they are relaxed and 'surrender' to the movement. With passive stretching, breathe in as you make contact and out as you apply the stretch.

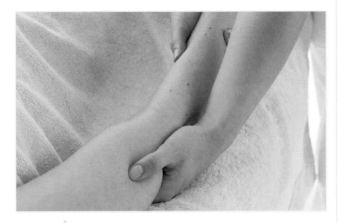

1 Use your inside hand to support your client's, resting it lightly on top of yours. With your outside hand, make contact just above the wrist, hand cupped around the outer edge of the arm with the thumb on top of the forearm. Apply pressure with the thumb pad and move up the arm to just below the elbow before rotating the wrist as before and gliding down the outer edge to the starting point, ready to repeat.

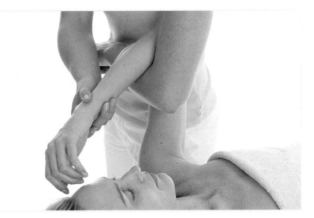

1 Positioning yourself at shoulder level, take the client's wrist with your inner hand and move the lower arm so it is at right angles to the upper arm. Place your outer arm under the crook of the elbow joint so that your inner elbow is against your client's as though you are linking arms. Using your body weight, lift your client's arm upwards off the table until you reach a point of resistance, then return it gently, ready to repeat if required.

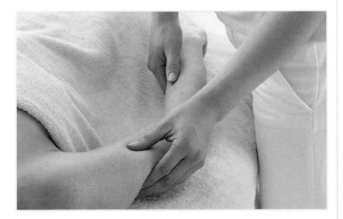

2 Slide your inside hand forwards to support your client's arm under the inside of the elbow, allowing their hand to rest lightly on your forearm. Using your outside hand, work deeply up the length of the bicep muscle from just above the elbow, kneading and squeezing this fleshy area. Glide down the outside edge of the arm, returning to the start.

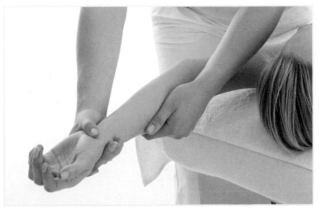

2 Still working on the same arm, take hold of the client's wrist as before, but this time lift the arm above the client's head, along the table as far as it will comfortably go. At the point of resistance, very gently give a slight pull from the wrist, taking care not to overextend the muscle, before gently placing the arm back alongside the torso.

Working the shoulder joint and arm

After draining and stretching the arms you are in a natural position to work on the shoulder joint. This ball and socket joint needs to maintain a wide range of movement, enabling further articulations of the arms and hands, but it sometimes gets neglected in a massage routine. You will need very little oil for this movement, ensuring that your hands do not slip off the area.

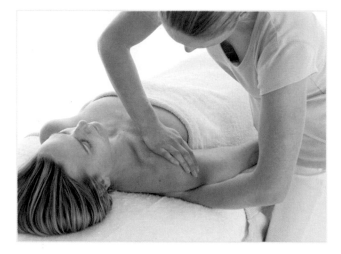

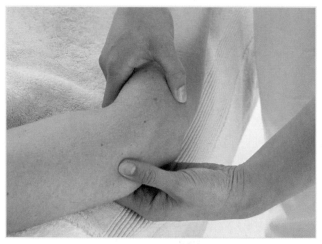

1 Positioning yourself alongside the client's elbow, lift the shoulder with both hands, putting your outer hand beneath the scapula, the tips of the fingers on the edge of the spine and the inner hand resting on the upper chest, below the collarbone. Sandwiching the torso between both hands, apply pressure and slowly pull both hands simultaneously off the edge of the shoulder. Repeat as required.

2 On the final shoulder joint movement, as your hands reach the edge, instead of sliding off, rotate them over the tops of the arms and work down the length of the arm to the elbow. Work around the joint using thumb and finger pads to apply friction to the muscle surrounding the bone before gliding down the forearm back to the wrist.

Working the wrist and hand

As the hands are the parts of the body that are most accustomed to touch, clients usually find this part of a massage extremely relaxing. It can also be a good way to finish a treatment, though you can massage the wrists and hands in almost any situation. It is useful when used as part of palliative care, on the elderly or in the workplace to maintain mobility. As with the shoulder joint, very little oil is required and you may wish to substitute a nourishing hand lotion for your usual massage medium.

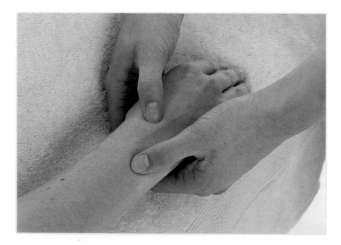

1 Take your client's hand using both of your hands, the fingers supporting the wrist and heel of the hand, leaving your thumbs free. Using your thumb pads, make contact over the bony area of your client's wrist and using circling strokes, slowly work over and in between the carpal bones along width and length. At this point of the sequence, you can slide your hands further down the hand and circle over the back of the hand, finishing at the web between the thumb and forefinger.

    If your client is pregnant, avoid the area in the web of the hand containing the powerful acupressure point called the Great Eliminator, as this is contraindicated.

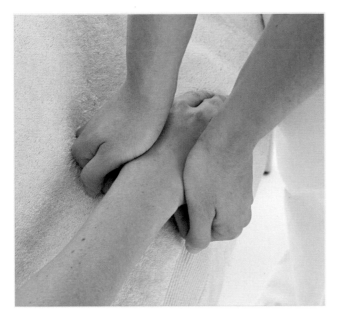

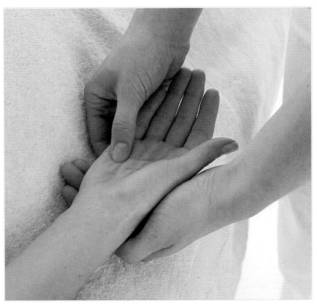

2 Returning to the wrist position, bring your thumbs alongside your fingers, sliding the heel of both hands on to the back of the client's. Applying downward pressure, glide both heels of hands firmly away from each other to the edges and return, ready to repeat. This will open up the palm of the hand and stretch out the whole area.

3 Turn the hand over, palm up and support the underneath with both hands as before, leaving the thumbs free to work. Using the thumb pads apply downward pressure and thumb circle over the whole palm. Continue circling down the fingers, at the same time squeezing the soft tissue surrounding the phalanges between your thumb and finger pads. This stroke can be applied with one hand if preferred, the other maintaining contact as the support hand (as shown above).

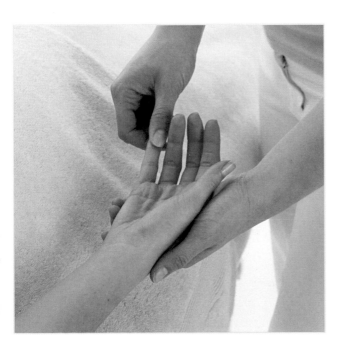

4 To finish off, clasp your client's hand with your outer hand and with the inner hand take hold of the tip of the little finger between the pads of your thumb and forefinger. Give it a gentle pull and shake, stretching out the finger and then release. Repeat on each finger and thumb in turn. This move would be contraindicated for any client with joint problems or arthritis. Substitute it by sandwiching their hand in between both of yours and gliding off slowly.

Working the front of the torso

The torso is divided into two main areas: the chest area, which includes the ribcage that protects all the major organs, and the abdomen, a vulnerable area of soft, unprotected muscle encasing the intestines, solar plexus and the area known in oriental medicine as the 'hara' or energy centre.

If starting a treatment with this area, be aware if its sensitivity and the need for your client to feel comfortable. Apply long, wide strokes rather than small, focused ones if your client is ticklish over the ribs and abdomen, using a firm touch.

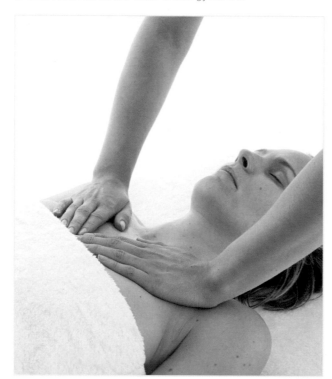

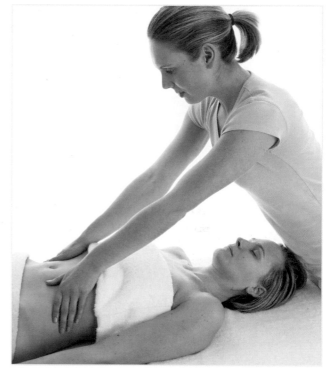

1 Position yourself at the head of the table, place your hands palm down on the middle of the upper chest and effleurage slowly down the centre of the torso, following the natural contours of the body. Avoid the breast area by placing one hand on top of the other and working through the centre. When you reach the navel, glide the hands outwards and return down the sides of the torso, pulling back slightly until returning to the upper chest, ready to repeat. A female client may wish to have the breast area covered with a small towel, in which case you will need to adapt the length of the stroke.

2 Repeat the above stroke, but instead of returning straight up the edge of the torso, move the hands simultaneously in large circles, slowly moving up the length of each side. After repeating three to five times, finish with your hands in the starting position on the upper chest.

Working the ribcage and chest

The broad, flat pectoral muscles that lie across the front of the chest wall and connect to the ribs not only have a protective role but also assist respiration.

The large diaphragm muscle and ribcage need to maintain flexibility to allow unrestricted breathing. Massage maintains mobility and releases fatigue and tension from this area.

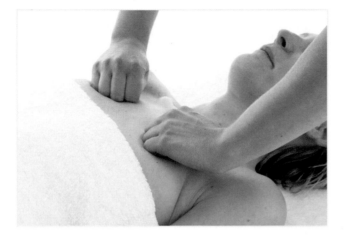

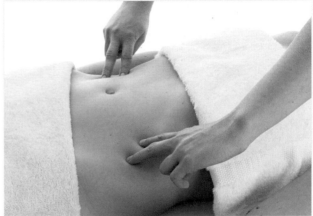

1 Following on from the long warm-up strokes, with hands positioned on the upper chest either side of the sternum or breastbone, make your hands into loose fists, facing each other. Make contact with the width of the knuckles and push them, both hands simultaneously, outwards against the soft tissue towards the armpits. Lift off and return to the centre. Repeat this movement in straight lines working down the chest. With a male client this can continue to the base of the ribcage, whilst women may feel more comfortable stopping on the upper edge of the breast.

2 Working the same area, with the index and middle finger of each hand forming a V shape and using the raking stroke, pull outwards from the top of the first rib along the bordering soft tissue to the sides. Work down the ribcage along each intercostal muscle, avoiding those directly under the breasts.

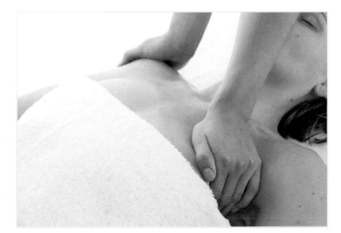

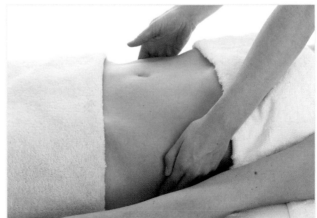

3 Resting one hand on a shoulder to maintain contact, place the heel of the other into the front of the corresponding pectoral muscle. This is the triangle of soft tissue lying alongside the armpit. Using petrissage, apply pressure through the heel of the hand, pushing through the soft tissue and off.

4 Using the flats of both hands in an alternate rhythm, make contact at the edge of the ribcage adjacent to the waist and, applying pressure, pull upwards and off, working along the side of the torso from the waist to the armpit. Repeat the last two strokes three to five times before reversing hands to repeat on the other side.

Working the abdomen

This sensitive area from the pelvis up to the bottom of the ribcage houses the important muscles that support the trunk and allow it to flex, rotate and tilt. Some clients may ask you to omit the abdomen from their massage because they are aware, usually subconsciously, that this is where emotional tensions are held and they are not ready to release them. This may be the case for a new client who needs to build up trust in you, so always ask permission before working on this area.

Take extra care where body piercing is present.

The golden rule for abdominal massage is to always move your hands in a clockwise direction, mimicking, rather than fighting the natural flow of the large intestine.

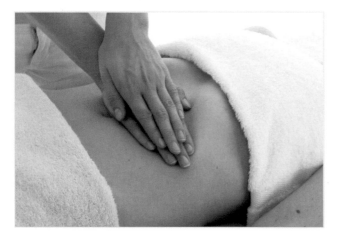

1 Working side-on, apply effleurage, one hand on top of the other, clockwise in sweeping circles over the whole area, working from the outer areas inwards. Start with gentle pressure, increasing as the size of the circles reduce. Apply the upper half of the circle on your client's inhalation, moving to the lower half on their exhalation.

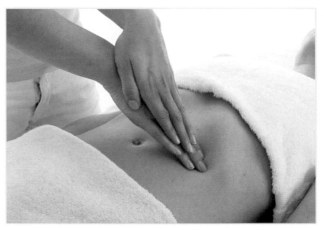

2 Keeping your hands on top of each other, raise up the heel of hand and using only the fingertips in a downward direction, make small rotations whilst tracing the large clockwise circles as before. Check your pressure with the client.

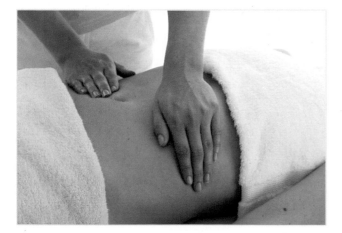

3 Place your hands palm down, either side of the abdomen and slightly cupped over the sides of the torso. Apply pressure through the hand nearest you, pushing outwards across the abdomen whilst at the same time pulling the other hand towards you, crossing in the centre. This movement needs to be firm but slow as you work up the entire length of the abdomen rhythmically.

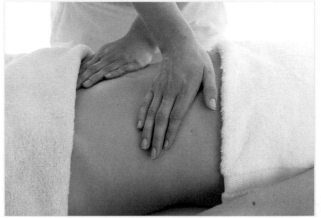

4 Finish the abdomen routine with an effleurage stroke to calm the area. Make contact on the lower edge of the abdomen centrally. Glide slowly upwards to the edge of the ribcage, lifting off slowly, fingers first, followed by the heel of hand. As one hand lifts off, make contact with the other hand at the starting position and follow through.

Working the front of the legs

The muscles of the lower limbs work hard; they are used almost constantly to walk, run, stand up and sit down. Tension is often stored in the muscles of the legs and feet which can hinder the pressure that is usually distributed evenly along the leg. This transference of force can cause painful conditions. For example, tightness of the adductor muscles in the upper leg can cause alterations to walking or running which may lead to sacro-iliac, hip or knee problems.

Regular massage maintains the elasticity of the muscles and helps to break down any adhesions. In sports massage, treatment of the legs is a major part of any pre and post event activity.

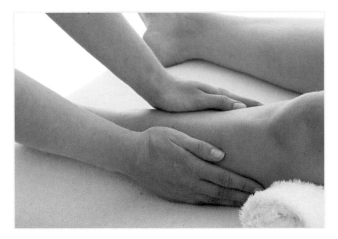

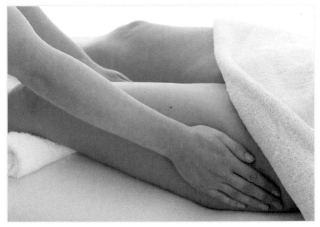

1 Position yourself facing up the table, in line with your client's ankles. Make contact with both hands and apply flat-handed effleurage along the topside of the leg. When you reach the knee joint, glide over the joint, lifting off any pressure, before continuing up the thigh, pushing into the muscle.

2 When you reach the top of the thigh, the outside hand can travel up as far as the hip, whereas the inside hand should remain at a level that is unintrusive. Rotate your wrists, allowing both hands to curve around the sides of the leg, ready to glide downwards to the start. If your arms and range of movement fall short of the length of stroke required, do not be tempted to push your elbows outwards to compensate for a long reach, simply position yourself slightly higher up the table to enable you to massage the whole leg.

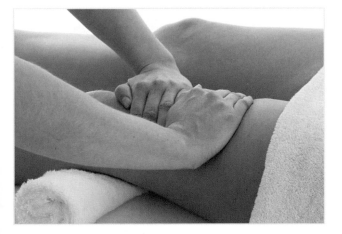

3 Repeat the above stroke along the length of the leg, this time using cupped instead of flat-handed effleurage. Make contact on the lower leg with both hands cupped and facing opposite directions. Glide up to the knee, using only light pressure over the shin bone, and as before, exert no pressure over the knee joint. Carry on up the thigh, which benefits from firm deep strokes, before returning down the sides as before.

Leg stretching

Legs respond well to passive stretching, which helps to exercise the hinge joints of the ankle and knee and the ball and socket hip joint and relaxes the leg for further work.

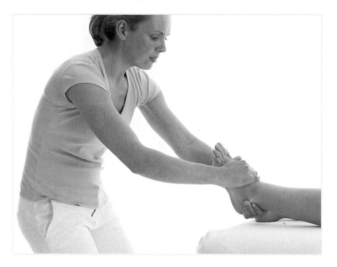

Place one hand across the top of the foot and with the other cup and support the heel, making sure your hold is firm and confident. Gently lift the leg upwards until it is raised a few centimetres above the table and then shift your weight backwards, pulling the leg slightly towards you, at the same time vibrating it very gently. Release the pull slowly before repeating once more, then gently return the relaxed leg to the table. To avoid overstraining, make sure that your pulling force comes from your body weight and not from just your arms and hands.

Working the knee and leg

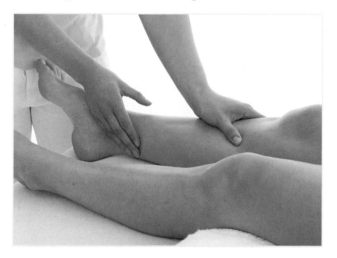

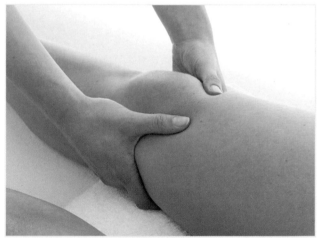

1 Place one hand above the ankle with the web of the hand in a V shape so that the thumb and finger pads are resting on the muscle either side of the shin bone. Push firmly along the muscle up to the edge of the knee joint and lift off whilst making contact with the other hand and following through hand over hand, repeating as required. This draining action will promote circulation and lymphatic drainage, but remember that ulcerated legs and working over and above varicose veins is contraindicated.

2 To work around the knee joint, place your hands under the knee for support, leaving the thumbs resting on the top of the leg. Using the thumb pads, move gradually around the outside of the knee pad from the top edge round to the bottom, pushing downwards and lifting along the natural groove. On each contact, maintain constant pressure for three to five seconds, making sure that your client is comfortable. Repeat the movement, this time rotating your thumb pads slowly instead of pressing downwards and lifting off until the whole knee cap has been circled. After working around the knee, continue up the thigh to the top of the leg using the strokes applied to the lower limb.

Working the hip joint and down the leg

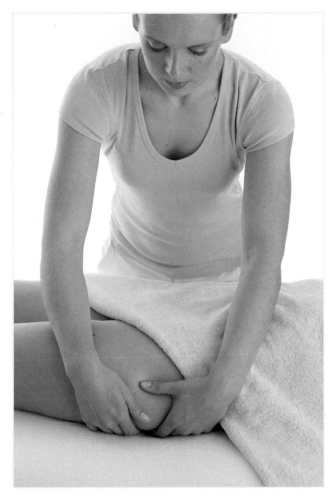

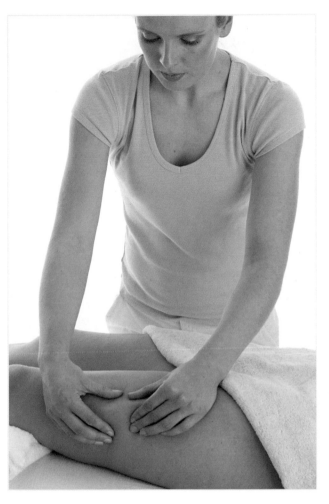

1 Position yourself side-on, level with your client's hip and make contact on the side of the gluteals just below the rim of the pelvis. Using the thumb rolling stroke, work around the hip joint, pushing deeply into the soft tissue that surrounds this large ball and socket joint.

2 With your hands palm down, tips of forefingers and thumbs slightly touching each other, press downwards and grab some muscle, 'rolling' it between your thumbs and fingers. Making sure that the skin is not pinched, work the front of the thigh and down the leg, gliding over the knee joint and working on the muscle either side of the shinbone to the ankle. As you move down the length of the leg, you will need to move your position smoothly down the table until you are at the foot of the table.

Working the front of the foot

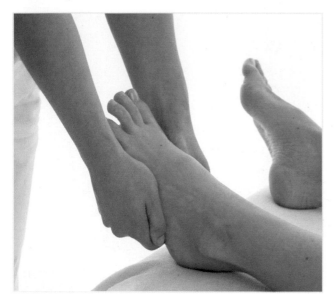

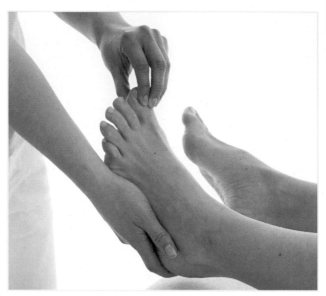

1 To complete the leg sequence, working with two hands, place the heels of the hands on the top of the foot, lean into your hands and glide them outwards towards the edge, firmly opening up the whole area. Make sure that your body weight is directly over the area, working with straight arms to avoid any strain or injury. If massaging with one hand, replace this stroke with a knuckling action, rotating the individual knuckles and the hand simultaneously, working over the top of the foot whilst supporting the underneath of the ankle with the other.

2 Still supporting the ankle, with the free hand take the base of the big toe between your thumb and finger and squeeze firmly. Gently pull the toe towards you, stretching it very slightly backwards and forwards, then slide your finger and thumb up the sides of the toe in a wringing action, releasing at the tip with a small squeeze and shake. Repeat this action on each toe.

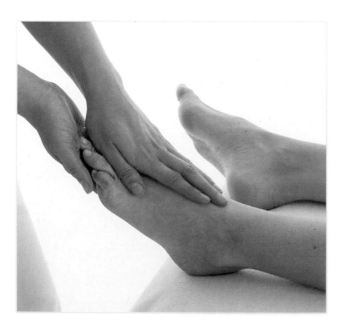

3 To finish off, sandwich the foot between the flats of your hands and apply effleurage, or with cupped hands work from the ankle over the top of the foot and back under the length of the sole.

Connecting and closing a massage sequence

Having learnt the basic strokes of massage and how to apply them on each section of the body you need to be able to 'bridge' areas together so that the client feels a sense of wholeness. The connecting and closing tools described here can be used between sections or at the end of the massage through towels to complete a treatment.

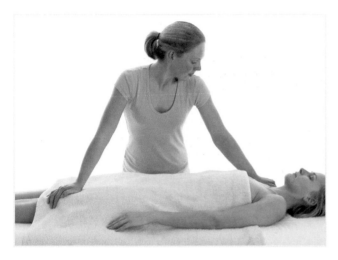

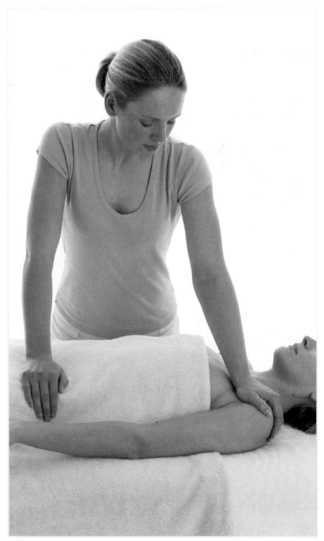

1 Position yourself side-on at a level that enables you to reach both the shoulder and down towards the foot in one long stroke. Place both hands on the navel and moving both hands simultaneously, glide one hand down the opposite leg and off near the foot, whilst gliding your other hand up the nearside of the chest and shoulder, down the arm and off at the hand. Return the hands to the navel and repeat on the opposite side.

2 Another method of connecting is the holding stroke, which can link any parts of the body and is easy to execute. Take the example of connecting the hip to the shoulder; simply place one hand on the hip and the other on the shoulder, palm down, and with gentle pressure hold the position for a few seconds, then lift off slowly and gently. As you commence a massage with 'contact' so you need to end with a 'connecting' hold.

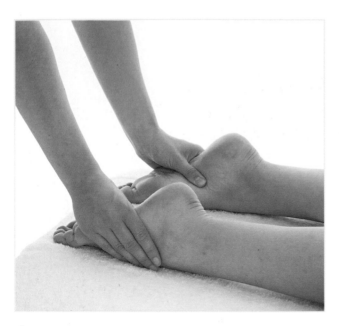

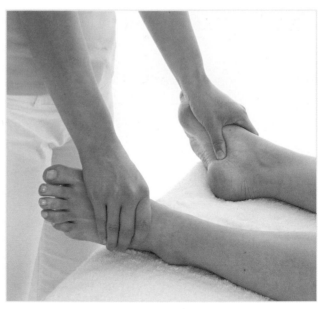

3 If you finish with the client prone, rest your hands on each foot with the thumbs placed on the insteps, apply medium pressure and hold for a few seconds before lifting off gently.

4 On a supine client, hold the feet over the tops and apply gentle pressure before lifting off gently.

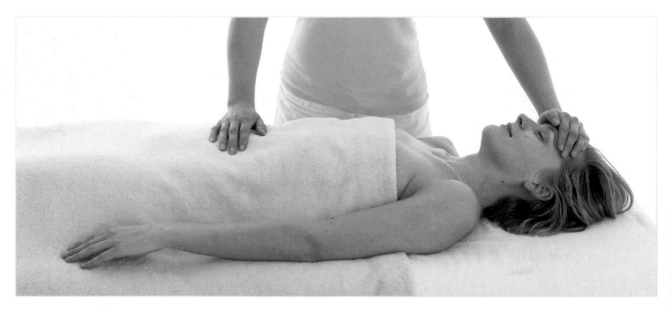

5 You may finish with a facial routine, in which case place one hand on the forehead and the other on the abdomen, holding for a few seconds before releasing slowly. This will allow the client to feel a connection between the head and the rest of the body so that the massage feels complete. A good massage should always have a definite beginning and end, so that the client does not leave with a sense that something was missing from the massage. These connecting and closing strokes will ensure a holistic treatment.

Aftercare

At the end of the treatment session, make sure that your client is fully covered with drapes and, unless they need help in returning to a sitting position and getting off the table, leave the room to let them to dress in privacy.

If you have applied oil or lotion to the feet, remind the client to use the towels to remove any excess to avoid a fall. Tell them you will meet them in the reception area in a few minutes and leave them a glass of water.

It is good professional practice to advise your clients that after a treatment they should drink plenty of water to speed up the flushing out of body toxins. Other effects could be headaches, thirst and frequent urination. After deep or friction work, the client may feel a slight 'sunburn effect' on the muscle area, which should disappear after 24 hours. They should be encouraged to telephone you if they are worried about any occurrences after receiving treatment.

Before your client leaves, check that they are fully aware and suggest they do not rush around for at least half an hour, letting the body return to normal.

It is also a good idea to obtain feedback at the end of the treatment about how your client is feeling, what areas they felt could have been worked on more or less, double check whether the pressure was comfortable and what they would like to happen on a following appointment. If a specific condition was being treated, you could call the client two or three days later to see if the problem has been alleviated. This is also useful when planning future treatments.

Checklist for 24-hour aftercare

Ensure that you advise the following to your client:

- Drink plenty of water.
- Avoid alcohol and strong stimulants for up to 12 hours.
- Encourage client to rest and not rush around.
- Take light meals, avoiding red meats where possible.
- Additional aftercare for specialized massage, e.g. sports or pregnancy massage, where applicable.

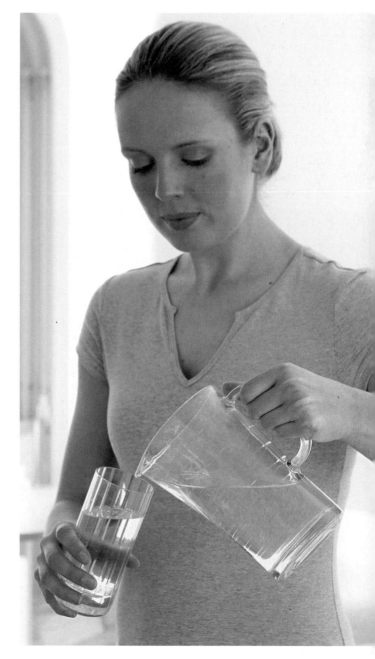

Water Offer your client a glass of water after each treatment and do not forget to drink plenty of water yourself between treatments to rehydrate the body.

Massage checklist

As a rough estimate a complete body massage will take between an hour and an hour and a half, but this timing is never rigid. It will depend on the needs of the client.

You may want to spend time focusing on an area of particular tension or at the request of the client, or there may be time constraints so you have to make a decision on what is important to include, for example back, neck and shoulders or face and scalp, chest arms and hands.

At the end of a shortened routine, use the long connecting strokes on the areas not massaged so that the client feels the whole body has been treated.

This basic Swedish massage routine is easy to understand and memorize and the one most commonly used. The back is often the area requiring the most work and focus and so the natural place to begin. When choosing a section to massage, always apply the basic rule of working towards the heart, applying pressure on the upward stroke, lighter on the return and lifting off pressure over joints and remember to work either side and not over the spine.

To build up confidence, particularly with a new client, you may decide to start slowly from the legs upwards, or to relax a very nervous or tense client start with the face. If it is a different routine from what they are used to, explain what you are going to do and why, so they feel comfortable. Tell them whether you would like them to lie prone or supine on the table to start the massage.

The following illustrations are a checklist of the routine, your working position, draping and the use of bolsters or pillows.

1 Contact

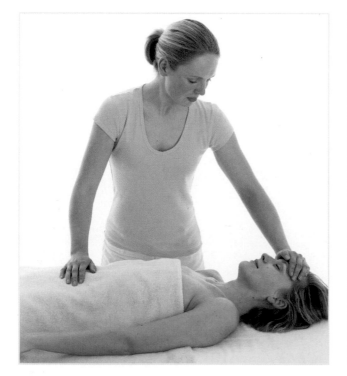

2 Back of body Upper back

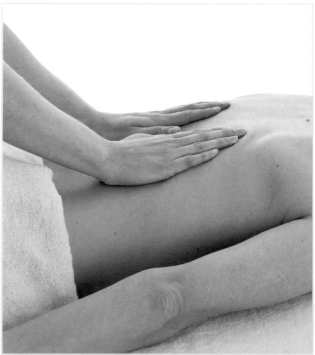

3 Back of body Spine

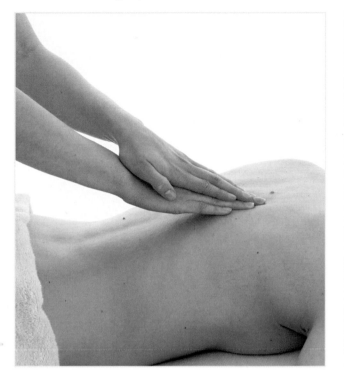

4 Back of body Lower back and buttocks

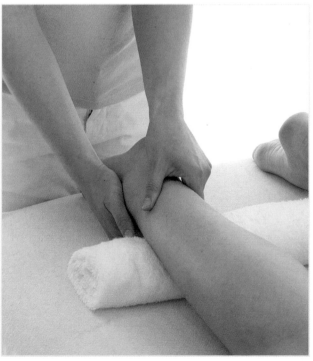

5 Back of body Backs of legs

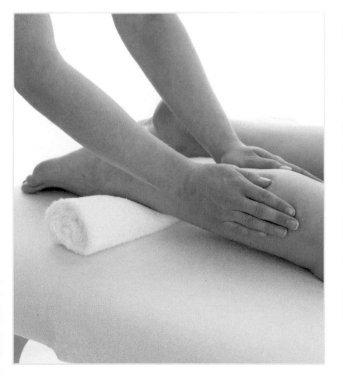

6 Back of body Ankle

7 Back of body Foot

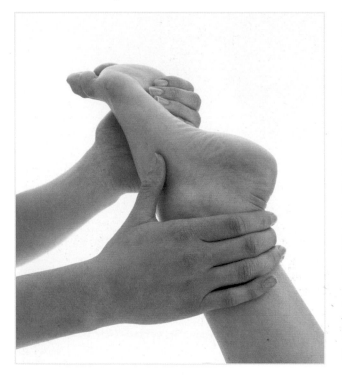

8 Front of body Shoulders, neck and scalp

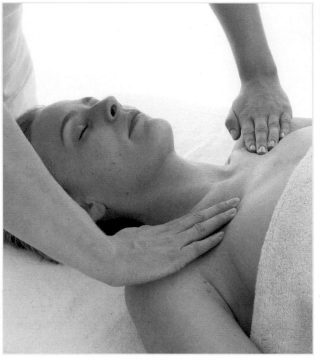

9 Front of body Face

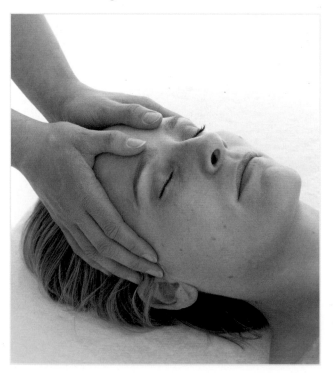

10 Front of body Arms and hands

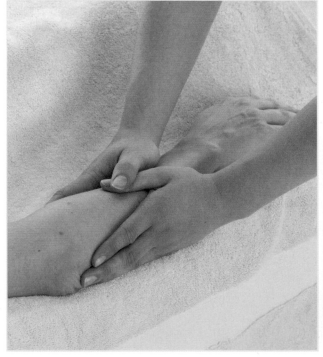

11 Front of body Chest and ribcage

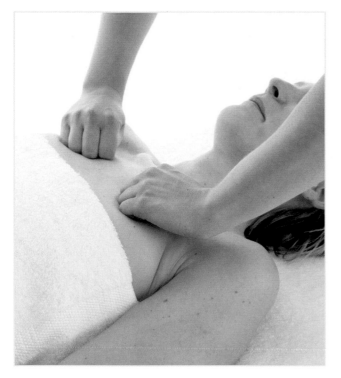

12 Front of body Abdomen

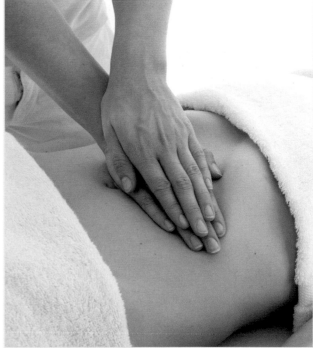

13 Front of body Front of legs and feet

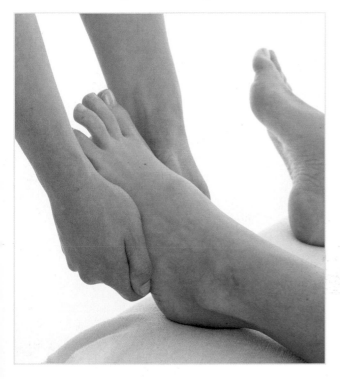

14 Finishing strokes

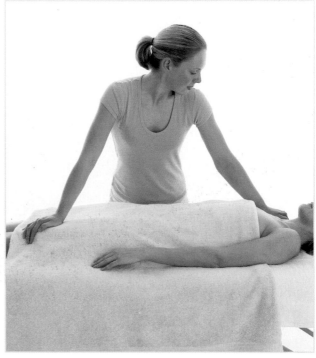

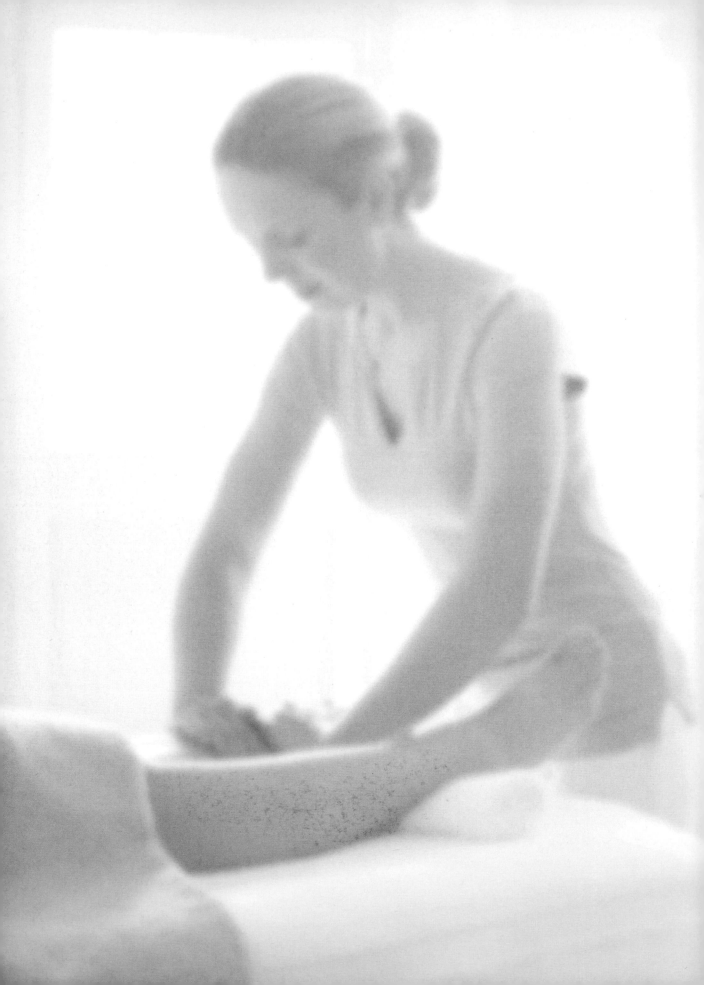

Specialized massage

At any stage of a person's life, human touch should play an integral part, from the start of life in the womb through to later years. Touch will help to promote well-being in times of good and poor health and provide the necessary relaxation to deal with the changes within our bodies at different stages of life. Massage is one way of ensuring that positive touch is received, using techniques that are adapted to specific conditions such as pregnancy, and for children of all ages, the elderly and those receiving palliative care.

Pregnancy

A healthy woman with a low-risk pregnancy is able to receive massage and all its benefits from the second trimester through to labour itself.

As the pregnancy progresses, the massage position will need to be adapted to keep the client comfortable, using several pillows for support. In the second trimester chair massage may feel more comfortable, but by the fifth month, getting the client to lie sideways with her stomach and upper leg supported with pillows is advisable. This position can also be used if massaging during labour.

Safety first

It is imperative that the following guidelines are observed when massaging a pregnant client:

- Do not massage during the first trimester or if the pregnancy is high risk (but see below).
- Avoid deep pressure and vigorous strokes.
- Avoid the abdomen, inner thigh and groin.
- Avoid pressure around and over the tops of the ankles.
- Up to the 36th week do not use essential oils in any form, even burning in the treatment room. Some oils are contraindicated for pregnancy so use pre-blended products designed specifically for pregnancy or consult a qualified aromatherapist.
- Do not massage if the physician disapproves of treatment during pregnancy.
- Do not massage if there is unexplained pain or discharge.
- Do not massage if nausea, vomiting or diarrhoea occurs.
- Leg massage is contraindicated if the client has poor circulation, severe oedema, is inactive or on bed rest.

Massage during the first trimester

During the first trimester of 14 weeks, the embryo grows to approximately 8 cm (3 in) and develops arms, legs, ears and nails. By day 26 an audible heartbeat can be detected. During this time the pregnant woman may suffer from headaches and fatigue due to hormone changes. Morning sickness may also occur and body temperature increases as the body becomes an 'incubator'. This is a very delicate time and although full body massage is contraindicated, head or face massage can be used to relieve anxiety and headaches.

Massage during the second trimester

From 14 to 28 weeks the baby grows to around 28 cm (11 in) long, develops eyebrows and lashes and becomes sensitive to light and sounds. The mother's body starts to change to accommodate the baby's growth; the ribs and pelvis move and as the body's centre of gravity changes, back pain may result. Massage using very light strokes can bring relief to indigestion and insomnia which are common at this stage.

Massage during the third trimester

From 28 to 40 weeks the baby increases in size and weight, the lungs are formed and sleep patterns develop. With the baby weighing an average of 2–4 kg (5–9 lb) at this stage, the mother noticeably increases in size, and moving and walking become more laboured. Conditions that may occur at this stage include heartburn, varicose veins, oedema in the legs, haemorroids and insomnia. Massage should be applied to the back, neck, shoulders and legs to relieve fatigue at this stage.

Massage during labour

The onset of labour is usually marked by the beginning of regular contractions, dilation of the cervix to 10 cm (4 in) and the rupture of the amniotic sac, often referred to as 'breaking waters'. This is followed by the actual birth or delivery of the baby and then the expulsion of the placenta or 'afterbirth'. During labour, massage of the lower back and buttocks can help the process to advance and may help with pain relief.

Positioning and bolstering during pregnancy

For the pregnant client you will need four or five standard size bed pillows as well as supports for the ankles and knees. If a large proportion of your work involves massage during pregnancy, you may want to consider investing in specialized pillow sets manufactured for the purpose. These pregnancy pillow systems are carefully designed to support the growing belly and lower back at the same time.

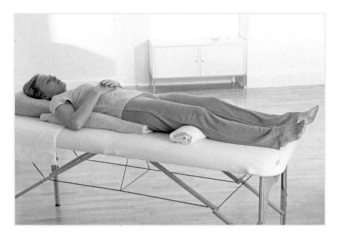

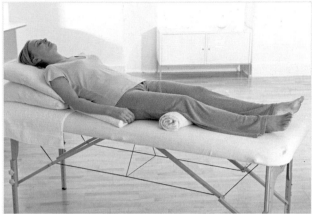

Left tilt

With client lying supine, place a small pillow or rolled-up towel under her right pelvis and torso in order to tilt the lower body to the left to avoid the uterus being pressed up against the spine. This will maintain the flow of oxygen and blood to the foetus.

Semi-seated

In the same position as the left tilt, support the client's upper body with pillows to a 45-degree angle in a semi-reclined stance. Use bolsters behind the knees and pillows under the lower arms for further comfort.

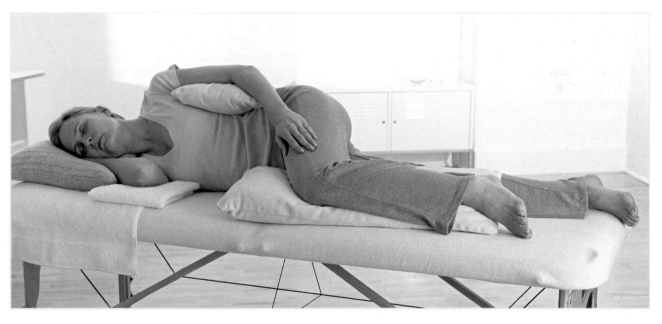

Side position

Using three or four pillows, ask the client to lie on her side with her back to the edge of the table. Place one pillow under her head, another under the upper arm away from the table, and a third supporting the knee and ankle. If the hip, knee and ankle are not in alignment, use a further pillow to attain the correct height.

Smaller pillows or rolled-up towels can be added for extra comfort between the wrist, ankle and abdomen resting on the table. Make sure the client is lying on the side they are most comfortable with, as they will remain in this position for most of the treatment.

Because all the work will be applied from a side position, your working stance will have to be adjusted accordingly and you may need to use a stool. Another option is to give the treatment on the floor in the final stages of a pregnancy.

CASE STUDY **PREGNANCY**

CLIENT PROFILE

Jennifer is seven months pregnant and in an age group where she is considered what is termed a geriatric mother – 43 years of age. Unlike the younger mothers she meets at her regular check ups, she finds that she has less energy and is finding it difficult to continue to work. In particular Jennifer is suffering regularly from lower back pain. Her company organizes a massage therapist to visit once every two weeks to offer treatments on a subsidised basis and the Human Resources department suggested that Jennifer book herself a treatment on the forthcoming visit.

REGULARITY

Providing that mother and baby are healthy and there are no contraindications, massage received once a week during the last two trimesters of a pregnancy will promote relaxation and bring relief to associated problems such as lower back pain and tired legs. Massage once a week during the second trimester, increasing to two a week, if possible, during the third would be most beneficial. They can range in duration from ten minutes, up to an hour.

TYPE OF TREATMENT

As the massage was performed by a visiting therapist on-site, a custom-made chair was available, enabling the massage to take place in a seated position, which was ideal for Jennifer. The therapist was able to access the lower back and top of the gluteals with ease. Other areas concentrated on were those compensating for Jennifer's shift in centre of gravity, such as the pectoralis major, lumbar spine and quadratus lumborum.

OUTCOME

The treatments brought some relief and Jennifer found a therapist close to home to visit alternate weeks so that she was able to receive a massage regularly. This enabled her to continue working until the start of her maternity leave and helped to keep her in good condition, ready for the birth, which is so important for any mother-to-be. She gave birth to a healthy baby girl.

Working the neck and lower back

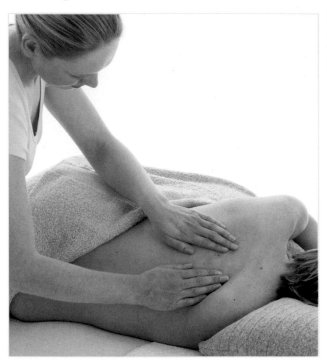

1 With your client lying sideways on the table, supported firmly under the stomach, position yourself at the side of the table facing up the table. Make contact either side of the spine on the lower back and using the flat-handed effleurage stroke, glide up the back to the top of the shoulders, returning down the sides of the torso, with pressure on the upward stroke only. Repeat three to five times.

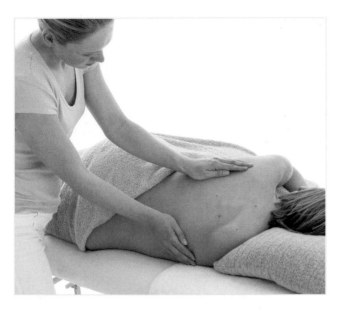

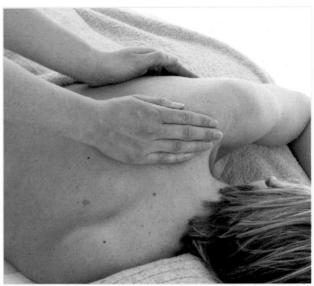

2 Work up the back as before, this time making small circles, hands working in opposite directions until you reach the top of the shoulders and return down the sides of the torso as before. Repeat three to five times.

3 Moving side-on to the table, working one side of the shoulder and then the other, place both hands at the base of the scapula, glide across the shoulder, then separate, returning one hand around the armpit and the other around the edge of the scapula, pulling back gently whilst returning to the start position. Repeat three to five times.

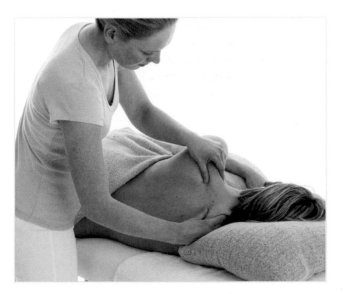

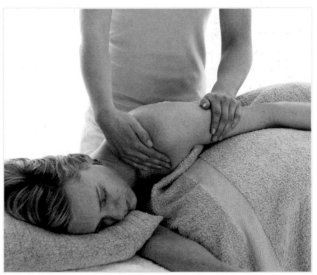

4 Place your hands on each shoulder and maintain contact for about 30 seconds, With your fingers positioned over the front of the neck and the thumbs at the back, squeeze the shoulder muscle between the heels of the hands and the fingers, working the length of the shoulder outwards to the tops of the arms and return. Repeat three to four times.

5 With hands on the front of the lower neck, fingers open, effleurage outwards from the sternum to the edge of the ribcage, using the pads of the fingers to massage the intercostal muscle of the upper ribs. Repeat the stroke three times before moving to the next intercostal space. Work the area from the top of the breast tissue upwards. This will help to open up the whole area, which often feels restricted and pressured during pregnancy.

Working the legs and ankles

As the pregnancy progresses, the legs become fatigued from carrying extra weight and altered posture. Massage, except where contraindicated, helps reduce water retention and any circulatory problems that may be present.

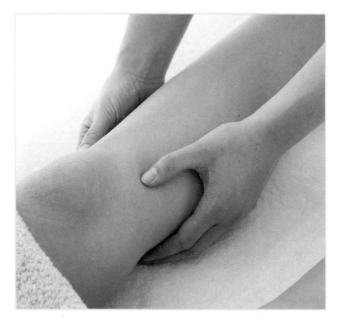

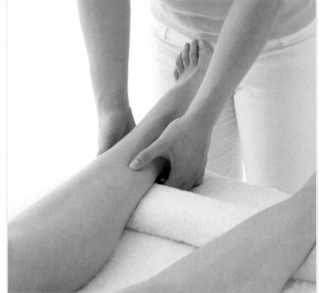

1 Make sure that your client is well supported and, positioning yourself at the end of the table, place the pads of both thumbs on the outer edges of the leg at the top of the shinbone, where it widens out towards the knee. Apply pressure through the thumb pads, pressing down three to five times. Check with the client that the pressure is comfortable.

2 Slide your hands down the leg, placing the thumb pads approximately four fingers width above the inner ankle. As before, apply pressure through the thumb pads, pressing down three to five times.

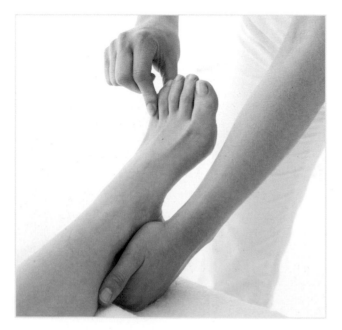

3 To finish the leg sequence, slide the hands down to the toes, support the base of the foot with one hand, take the small toe between your index finger and thumb and pull off in a downward movement, squeezing and rotating very slightly as you move down the length of the toe. Apply the same stroke to each toe in turn, before repeating the whole sequence on the other leg.

Babies and children

Massage is as beneficial for babies and children as it is for adults, and it also gives additional specific advantages, such as improving communication and bonding between parents and child.

Research shows that you are never too young to receive massage; it has been proved to encourage growth and development in babies, improve muscle tone and aid communication. Babies sleep and feed better with regular stoking and stretching during the first few months of life, and common infant conditions such as colic and constipation can also be relieved with specific techniques. Although massaging a baby or small child can be quite challenging, as they tend to move around and join in with the proceedings, it can also be extremely rewarding.

Massage therapists can legally treat children, but there is a legal responsibility in most countries for the parent or guardian to ensure the child has 'correct medical aid'. You must therefore check that a doctor has been consulted and inform the parents of this necessity. If you cannot be sure a doctor has been consulted, you are required to have the parents sign a statement saying they have been informed of their responsibility.

You should never conduct a physical examination of a child under 16 without the presence of a parent, guardian or responsible adult known to the child.

Children and teenagers

For children between the ages of 3 and 18 years of age, the massage to be applied should be explained during the consultation process to both parent or guardian and child.

To fulfil legal requirements there should be some supervision of the treatment. You should check the legal requirements pertaining to the country where you practise to make sure that you are complying with the law. If massaging a child or teenager of the opposite sex it would be prudent for both parties to make sure that a parent is present at all times.

When massaging adolescent males, extra caution is needed as sometimes a reflex sexual erection occurs when applying strokes to the thighs and abdomen. Be aware that the client will be more embarrassed and unprepared for this reaction than the therapist.

CASE STUDY **BABIES AND CHILDREN**

CLIENT PROFILE
John, an eight-month-old baby, seemed to cry excessively and his mother was at a loss what to do. There were no obvious signs of what may be causing the unrest and the baby was healthy. Bedtimes were becoming increasingly difficult and both mother and baby were very fatigued. A massage therapist was consulted to see if a relaxation treatment would help.

When a baby has experienced a traumatic birth, for example, a forceps delivery, there are sometimes emotional repercussions and cranial osteopathy may be recommended to address the situation.

REGULARITY
A programme of one massage a week for the first month was advised, to be followed by treatments as and when required. It was also suggested that the mother learn a few techniques to apply at home in between the professional treatments.

TYPE OF TREATMENT
Remembering to 'listen' to John and proceeding only with his co-operation, full body massage was applied where possible. On other occasions hands and feet or back were focused on. Simple effleurage and some light thumb rolling strokes were applied using a suitable carrier oil, sometimes mixed, by an aromatherapist, with lavender essential oil to promote relaxation.

OUTCOME
Within five minutes of the first treatment John was almost asleep much to the delight of his mother, who wondered why she had not introduced massage sooner and prevented months of unnecessary unrest.

SAFETY FIRST

It is imperative that the following guidelines are observed when massaging a baby:

- For babies four to six weeks old, before they have had their full health assessment, only apply light stroking. Thereafter a full massage sequence can be given.
- Wait for a week after any vaccination or immunization before massaging.

- Do not massage if there appear to be any unstable joints or brittle bones.
- Do not massage for at least one and half hours after feeding.
- Do not massage if the baby has any infection, skin rash or is medicated.
- Take extra care to avoid massaging directly on the spine.
- If a baby is born prematurely, only administer light stroking for the first four to six weeks.

Babies and toddlers

A treatment room used for massaging babies and small children will require extra attention. It should be kept very warm as babies lose body heat quicker than older children and adults. You should also make sure your hands are warmer than for massaging an adult. For a baby, use a changing mat covered with a clean towel on top of the massage table, or work with the baby on your knees or lap and keep spare towels to hand in case of 'accidents'. For your massage medium use a simple vegetable oil such as sunflower or a pre-blended massage (not baby) oil specifically for babies.

When you are ready to commence the massage, 'listen' to the baby or child and never proceed without full cooperation. All the strokes can be applied three to four times, depending on the response from the baby. The whole sequence should only last around ten minutes, unless the baby is calm and relaxed and happy for it to carry on longer. Stop when they indicate they have had enough and, as with adults and children, they may feel thirsty afterwards as the massage encourage the release of toxins and waste.

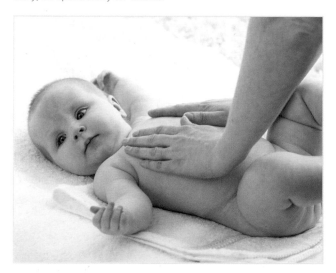

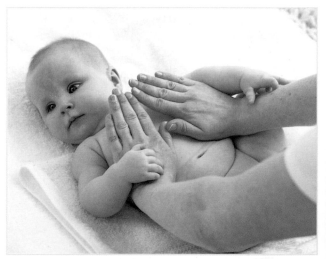

1 Sit in a comfortable position, with the baby facing you. Place the flats of your oiled hands on the centre of the chest and hold this position. Apply slight pressure and then slowly release it while still maintaining contact. Making the first touch in this way will reassure and relax the baby, preparing for the following strokes.

2 Keeping your thumbs in the centre of the baby's chest, use the heels of both hands to massage outwards and downwards around the lower ribcage and return. Repeat this three or four times.

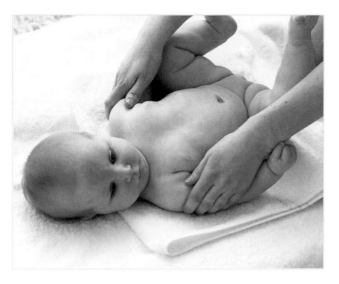

3 From the central position, and using the flat-handed effleurage stroke, massage upwards and outwards across the baby's shoulders and the tops of the arms, returning to the centre in one rhythmic sweep. Repeat this three or four times.

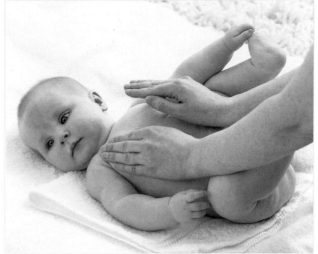

4 With your hands cupped slightly, use a percussion stroke to work lightly across the top and sides of the chest. Continue this for 15 seconds.

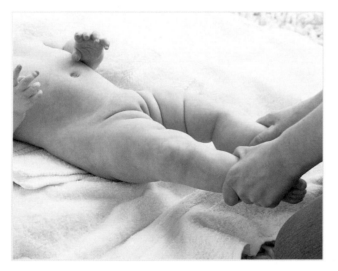

5 Using both hands from the central position, effleurage upwards and outwards across the baby's shoulders and the tops of the arms again. Return to the centre and continue down the trunk to the legs and feet. Without breaking contact, continue to work back up the body in reverse and finish by stroking down each arm. This should be one long sweeping stroke. Repeat this three or four times.

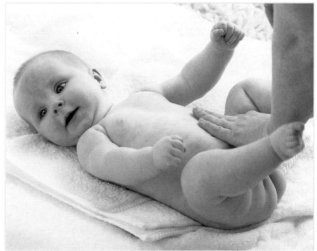

6 Using the fingers of one hand, stroke diagonally from the top of the baby's shoulder to the opposite hip. As you reach the end of your stroke, lift your other hand, ready to repeat the movement on the other side. Imagine you are drawing an invisible X across the front of the chest, using your hands alternately. Repeat this three or four times.

Elders

The elderly or geriatric population, generally considered to include anyone over 70 years of age, is the fastest growing section of the community. An elderly person can still be sprightly and independent, whereas another of the same age may be quite frail and need assistance or skilled help.

Massage can play an important role in keeping an elderly person healthy and supple, and in some cases it can re-introduce caring 'touch' into their lives.

The body changes physically in a variety of ways as we age: the nerve and reflex actions are slower and because of the effect on the nervous system there may be a loss of sensitivity to pain. Sometimes the opposite occurs and there is an increased sensitivity. The senses in general are affected, with reduced hearing and eyesight being common. As the anatomy and physiology deteriorates, flexibility and muscle tone decreases, bones and joints are not as strong and the skin starts to thin. The speed at which these degenerative processes occurs often depends on how mobile and active the person is. In a sedentary lifestyle circulation is poor, which will encourage lack of mobility and loss of muscle tone. This also tends to result in incontinence as the urinary and gastrointestinal tracts become more flaccid.

When massaging the elderly, deep work is usually contraindicated unless the physician feels it would be beneficial. Gentle passive stretching is encouraged but mobilizations, particularly of the neck, are not suitable because of the increased fragility of the skeletal system.

You will also need to build extra time into the massage sessions, as they may take longer to dress and undress, and may also want to share some conversation time with you.

If you are visiting the client in a residential or nursing home, make sure that your treatment is consistent with what you would give a client living in their family home or at a clinic. Always knock on the door of the room before entering and leave the room as you have found it.

Massaging the elderly often requires particular sensitivity and patience. If you do not feel able to adapt to this, refer clients to a therapist who specializes in this area.

Simple massage routine for the elderly

This simple seated routine does not require the removal of clothes or use of oils, but is a great pick-me-up.

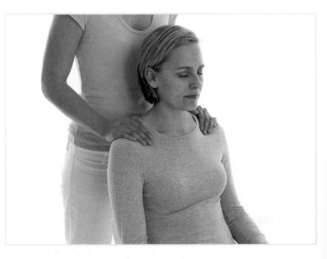

1 Make sure the client is seated in a comfortable chair that does not have a high back. Stand or sit behind the chair and make contact by resting a hand on each shoulder. This will enable you to sense the tension stored and whether the client is relaxed or not. Encourage them to let go of their thoughts, close their eyes and enjoy the experience.

AFTERCARE

Elderly clients will often feel light-headed or dizzy when returning to a sitting position after lying down on a massage table. This is due to a sudden drop in blood pressure. The therapist should be aware of this and assist the movement, making sure they are feeling fine before helping them to their feet.

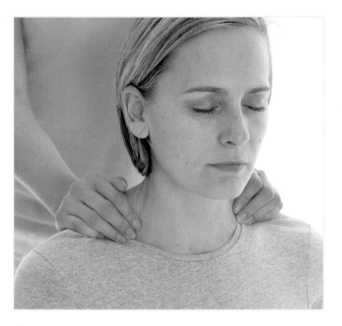

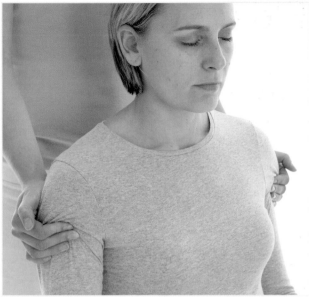

2 With fingers forward over the tops of the shoulders, using the heels of the hands and the thumbs, apply a petrissage stroke, squeezing the muscle and working along the top of the shoulder. Increase the depth and pressure of stroke where required, making sure the client is comfortable.

3 Continue the petrissage over the top of the shoulder and down the upper arms to just above the elbow joint before returning to the base of the neck.

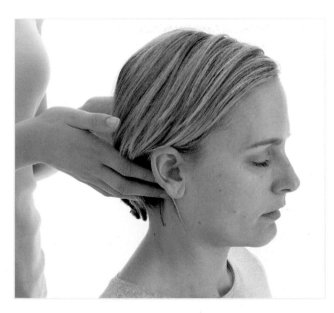

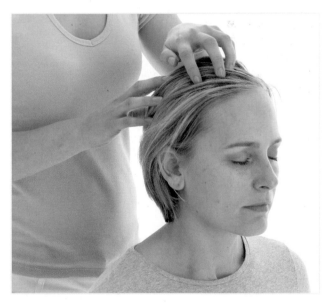

4 Cup your hands behind the neck and using the pads of the fingers apply pressure, working in small circles either side of the neck, up to the base of the skull. Making sure that your fingers are not on the neck or head, place the finger pads along the base of the skull, apply pressure and hold for five seconds before releasing. Rotate the pads of the fingers, applying pressure at the same time and release.

5 To finish the sequence, comb your fingers lightly through the hair to the top of the head. Place your hands back on the shoulders, hold for a few seconds and lift off.

Palliative care

The dictionary definition of palliative is 'relieving without curing', which could be applied to all types of massage. However, the term is usually used when describing massage for people who have a chronic or terminal illness and may be in hospital or a hospice.

A chronic illness is one with no known cure, for example, multiple sclerosis, lupus, fibromyalgia or Parkinson's disease, whereas a terminal illness is a condition that has a definite time frame. The aim of massage in both cases is to improve the quality of life as far as possible.

The main modifications you will need to make when writing your treatment plan for a client with a chronic or terminal illness is not in the strokes themselves, but in how they are applied. The pressure, pace and duration of the strokes, length of the session and how the client is positioned on the massage table, together with specific safety precautions all need to be considered. The client may also have certain demands to be incorporated. It is important that you learn about the condition and its pathology before a treatment, and most of all, you should be patient, open minded and flexible.

Clients in this category will usually have good and bad days with widely varying tolerances and responsiveness to touch. Each massage session will be very different and may produce a variety of emotional responses. Before agreeing to massage, medical clearance is usually necessary and the treatment plan itself should be for shorter periods and gentler in pace and pressure than that for a healthy client. Some passive stretching and mobilization work may help if the client feels well enough,

Palliative care massage
Massage during palliative care may be restricted to a gentle hand or foot massage where the focus is entirely on the person and their comfort.

as it provides 'exercise' for weakened limbs and muscle tone, but the massage may be very tiring and so should be monitored with constant feedback from the client.

Massage in palliative care is the one exception to the rule about not massaging on a regular bed. For the bedridden client only gentle hand or foot massage may be possible and in these circumstances it will be more comfortable and practical for them to remain in bed. If visiting a client in hospital, check with the nursing staff for any specific contraindications and work carefully around equipment.

Massage for the patient with HIV/AIDS

A condition you may come across as a therapist if you are providing massage for clients in palliative care is HIV/AIDS, a disease that affects the immune system and can be transmitted through contact with body fluids.

These days, with modern anti-retroviral drugs, a person infected with the HIV virus can live for many years without developing AIDS.

Although it is safe to massage a client with HIV or AIDs, and there has never been a case recorded of a therapist contracting it from a client and vice versa, there are some simple guidelines that should be observed. The immune system of the client may be low and you have a responsibility to make sure that your cleanliness is sufficient to reduce the risk of exposing your client to infection. Do not agree to a massage if you are suffering from a cold or other virus and make sure that any wounds, however small, have healed or are covered.

It may be necessary to adapt your treatment plan according to the client's condition on the day of your visit. For example, if they are tired, apply gentle massage for a shorter duration. Observe contraindications as you would with any other client, avoiding lesions, sarcoma, or recent locations of injections or transfusions.

If the client has not disclosed this condition on their initial consultation, but you suspect that they are HIV-positive or living with AIDS, you are not permitted to ask if they have the condition.

The final days

If you are called to massage a client who is in the last stage of their life, you will need to prepare yourself and your feelings about death and dying. Massage can really help reduce suffering and make the client comfortable. It should help them not to feel isolated or lonely and is a way to communicate without verbalizing, which is sometimes difficult. The touch should be calming and reassuring. You will need to be very focused as it is a great personal commitment.

CASE STUDY **PALLIATIVE CARE**

CLIENT PROFILE
Ian had a stroke two years ago when he was just 49 years old. Going to work one morning he felt a little strange and had noticed a slight change to his face when trying to shave that morning. His co-ordination was poor, but he struggled to catch the bus and on arriving at work was told immediately to go to hospital as he was not well. He was diagnosed as having had a cerebrovascular accident, which had resulted in a slight loss of function of the voluntary and involuntary muscles in the right side of the body. As part of his on-going therapy, massage was suggested.

REGULARITY
Initially massages were given regularly but were short in duration in order to promote the reduction in spasticity and also provide emotional support. Whilst recovering under medical supervision, these were available daily. However, Ian felt they were very beneficial and continued to have massage once a fortnight on returning home, reducing to once a month in the long term.

TYPE OF TREATMENT
The massage focused on the right side of the body, both upper and lower limbs, starting proximally and ending at the foot or hand. Effleurage, petrissage and friction were applied with great care as Ian was not able to give feedback on the pressure, due to the loss of sensation. The pressure was gradually increased with each treatment, making sure that the limbs were well supported at all times. As Ian's left side (unaffected) was very tense due overworking, massage was applied to the left neck, shoulder and upper body to help reduce stress and relax the muscles.

OUTCOME
Two years later Ian has recovered much of the sensation he initially lost and is able to lead a 'normal' life. He has returned to work in a less stressful role and continues to have regular massage as it helps him to keep stress at a manageable level and gives him an awareness of his general body condition.

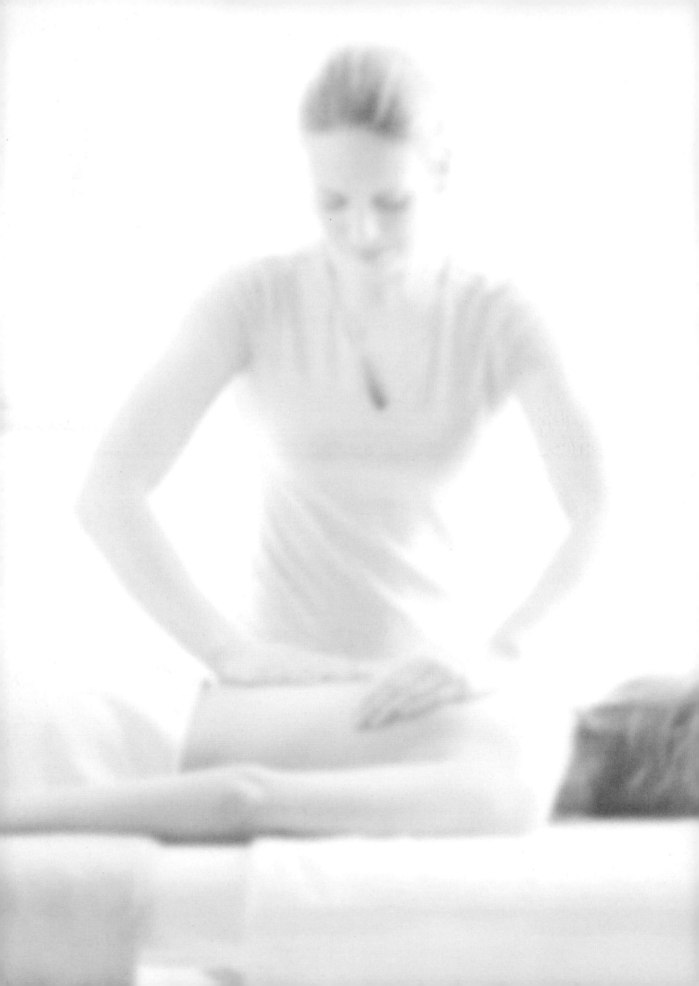

Massage for common ailments

Over the last 25 years massage has risen in popularity as a supplement to medical treatments and to prevent and maintain well-being. In our modern, highly pressured lives, the prevalence of conditions related to stress and anxiety has grown enormously, and many of these respond particularly well to massage therapy. In this chapter we look at a few common ailments that you are likely to come across when treating clients and provide detailed step-by-step descriptions of suitable massage routines.

Insomnia

Often a side-effect of stress or anxiety, insomnia is an inability to sleep or to stay asleep for a whole night. Sleep deprivation can have serious long-term effects on the body. Lack of sleep can become habitual and needs to be addressed as it can promote feelings of irritability, anxiousness and even depression.

The sleep required by the body depends on age: babies need around 17 hours a day, whereas adults need seven or eight. A number of factors other than stress and anxiety can contribute to insomnia, including physical health problems causing pain or poor respiration, environmental issues such as temperature, outside noise or poor bedding.

Jet lag following long-haul flights and lifestyle choices including late night eating and drinking can also affect sleep patterns.

Insomnia is classified into two types: primary insomnia has an underlying cause that is obvious, and secondary insomnia caused by medication or substance abuse. Primary insomnia is thought to account for a third of cases and secondary insomnia is responsible for a fifth.

Massage can help in the case of transient or short-term insomnia by promoting natural sleep. For chronic insomnia, regular treatments may help to break the fatigue cycle that occurs through lack of sleep.

Use gentle, rhythmic strokes and encourage the client to empty their mind of the thoughts of the day.

Massage routine

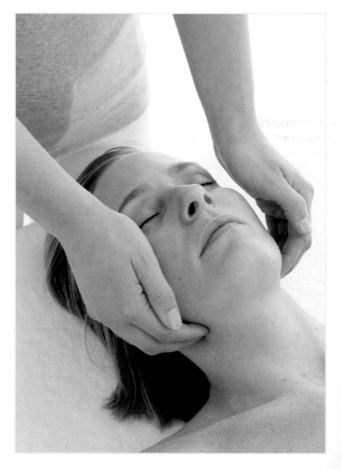

1 Position yourself at the head of the table with the client supine. Leaning forward, make contact by placing the fingers of both hands on the chin. Using the pads of the fingers, rotate in small circles, moving along the jawline outwards to just in front of the ear lobes.

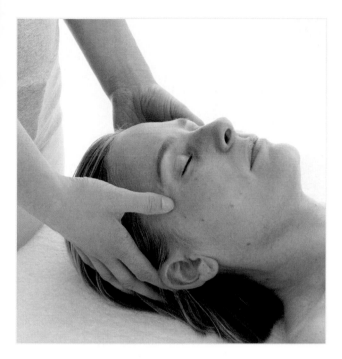

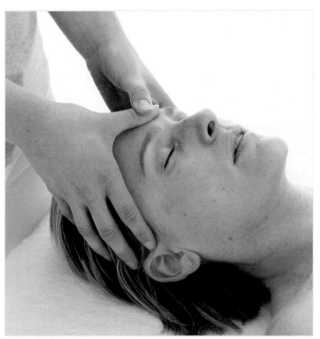

2 Place your thumbs together, making contact at the centre of the forehead. Place the rest of your hands either side of the skull in alignment with the hairline. Glide each thumb outwards, working towards the temples, lift off and return to the centre. Repeat this movement several times, each time placing the thumbs in a starting position higher than the time before, until the whole forehead has been worked.

3 Position the thumbs, one on top of the other in a reinforced position at the centre of the forehead close to the hairline. Exert pressure, hold for a few seconds and release. Repeat, moving upwards and over the skull to the centre.

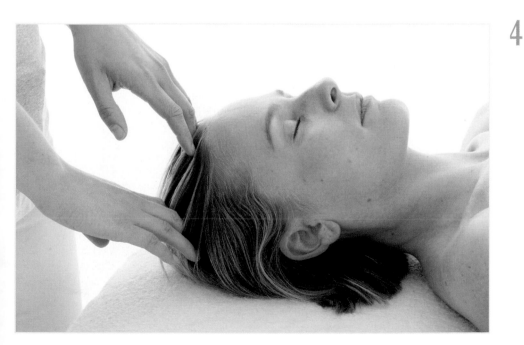

4 Using both hands in a combing action, fingers splayed, gently draw them through the hair, moving one hand and then the other in a continuous rhythmic action. This routine can be used at the end of a longer body massage or as a stand-alone treatment at the end of the day.

Headaches and migraines

Headaches, whether muscular, cluster, eyestrain, mental fatigue or sinus, respond well to massage. It is a common method of relieving migraines between attacks and can help reduce the frequency of headaches.

Headache manifests itself as pain at the base of the skull, the top of the head, the temples and the forehead and can be very debilitating. Chronic problems may benefit by referral to a chiropractor, but massage will bring general relief by stimulating the flow of blood to the brain.

Massage routine

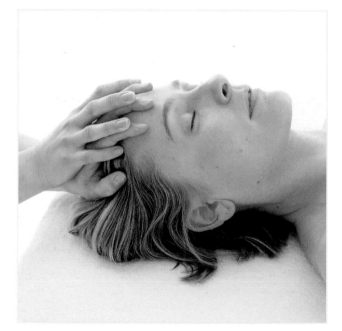

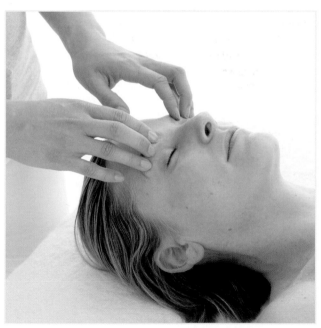

1 Position yourself at the head of the table and make contact by placing one hand, fingers spread, on the client's head and forehead. Gently place your other hand on top, slowly leaning into the hands. Check your client is happy with the pressure and hold for ten seconds before lifting off, but maintaining contact. Repeat three to four times. This movement is particularly effective for headache in the forehead region.

2 In the same working position, place your hands either side of the lower forehead with the finger pads on the brow bones. Hooking the tips of the finger pads along the underside of the brow bone, hold for ten seconds, then release, repeating three to our times. This area can be very sensitive so take care not to apply too much pressure.

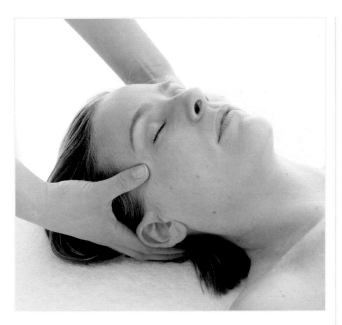

3 Still in the same position, slide your hands to the sides of the head, fingers behind the ear and thumbs positioned over the temples. Using the pads of the thumbs, rotate them slowly in a clockwise direction for ten seconds. This is a very small movement and the slower it is applied the more relaxing it will feel. Check that your client is comfortable and hold the pressure without rotations for ten seconds before lifting off.

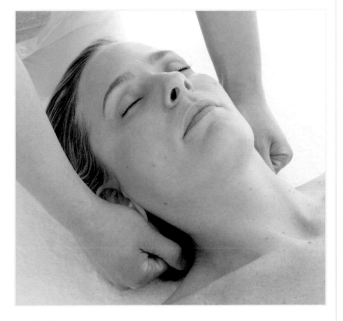

4 To finish, bring the heel of your hands down to cover each ear, curl your fingers underneath and draw your hands down and off.

Sinus headaches

Sinus headaches are caused by congestion or inflammation of the cavities that drain into the nasal passages. The sinus area becomes painful, heavy and uncomfortable. Infection of the sinuses can be caused by pollution or the presence of bacteria.

Massage routine

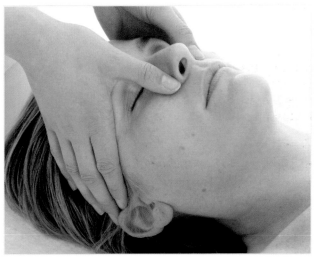

1 Place the thumbs of each hand either side of the bridge of the nose, ask your client to breathe in, on the out breath glide the pads of the thumbs simultaneously down the sides of the nostril and under the edge of the cheekbones, following the natural channel. Repeat several times.

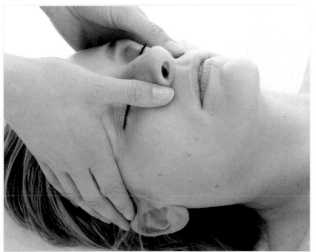

2 With the pads of the thumbs, work down the sinus tracts palpating the area to encourage drainage.

Tennis elbow

This common condition is associated with racket games, particularly when played strenuously. It is caused by tightening and overstraining of the wrist extensors or can also be the result of nodules or lesions that make the muscles vulnerable to injury.

The medical term for tennis elbow is lateral epicondylitis. It is caused by inflammation of the tendons in the forearm, near the elbow. The first indication of a problem is a dull ache in the mid section of the forearm that occurs each time there is wrist or arm action. Deep-friction massage and some joint mobilization will bring relief, but if chronic, the wrist should be totally rested to allow healing; otherwise, aggravation could rupture the tendon.

You do not have to be a tennis player to suffer from tennis elbow; using a computer mouse and keyboard, playing instruments, such as the violin, or manual work that involves repetitive twisting and lifting motions can also result in the condition. Gentle warm-ups before activity and regular breaks will help to prevent it.

Massage routine

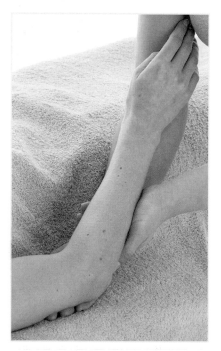

1 Rest the client's underarm on your forearm, supporting the elbow in the cup of your hand.

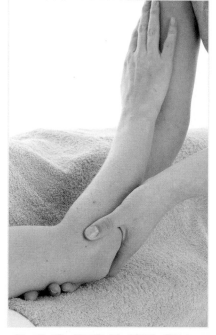

2 With the pad of your thumb positioned on the outside elbow and the fingers underneath to apply counter pressure, work in small circles around the outside of the elbow.

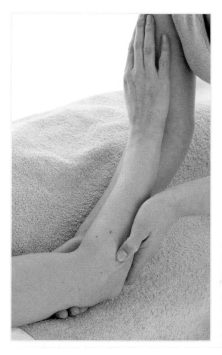

3 Keeping your hands in the same position and using the tip of the thumb, not the pad, apply pressure in a back and forth movement across the elbow in a cross-fibre technique.

Indigestion

Digestive problems are often linked with state of mind. Stress can manifest itself in conditions such as stomach ulcers, constipation or diarrhoea.

Because stress inhibits the flow of blood to the digestive tract, it can affect the passage of food through the tract and the absorption of nutrients. It can also affect the distribution of nutrition around the body.

Indigestion is a term used for any difficulty, pain or discomfort that occurs when ingesting food. Massage applied to induce relaxation and stimulate the blood and lymph flow will help to restore the digestive process to normal.

The abdominal area is one of the most sensitive and unprotected parts of the body, which is why clients are often averse to having massage applied here. Whether you believe, as some do, that emotions are stored in the abdomen, it is clear that the stomach and the emotions are closely linked, as shown by the use of phrases such as 'butterflies in the stomach' or 'my heart was in my stomach'. Because of this relationship it is necessary to treat abdominal massage with extra care and sensitivity.

Massage routine

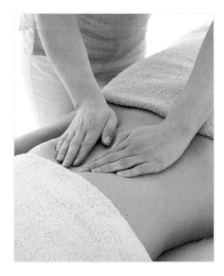 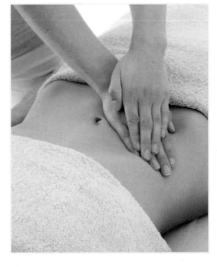 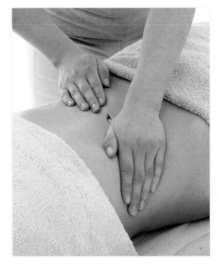

1 With the client supine, make contact on the lower torso with both hands, and using flat-handed effleurage glide upwards to just under the breast area. With your hands either side of the torso, slowly return to the starting position. Repeat this movement five times smoothly and gently. The aim is to calm and soothe. This is very beneficial for bloating and indigestion.

2 Place one hand on top of the other in the reinforced effleurage position. Working in a circular clockwise direction, gently travel the hand from the area of the solar plexus, following the direction of the large intestine. Begin with a large sweeping circle, gradually reducing the size of the circles, but increasing the pressure applied. Make four or five rotations and follow the breathing pattern with your hands.

3 Once the area has been warmed up and relaxed, place the hands facing each other and applying gentle pressure: on the client's outbreath, draw the hands apart diagonally; for example, right ribs to left hip. Work outwards in a sweeping action and repeat in the other direction. The aim is to stretch rather than work deeply in order to aid the release of any contracted muscle.

Asthma

Asthma is one of the common symptoms of respiratory stress. It has become increasingly prevalent in the modern world because of poor air quality, the use of domestic and industrial chemicals and pollution.

In an asthma attack, spasm and inflammation of the respiratory tract causes difficulties in breathing and tightening of the chest muscle. Asthma cannot be cured by massage, but treatment may reduce the frequency of attacks. The severity of the condition is sometimes related to emotional states caused by stress and anxiety, and this is when massage can be very beneficial.

Remember to relax and warm the localized area to be worked with gentle effleurage before applying deeper techniques. Massage would not be appropriate during an unrelenting asthma attack, where infection is present or if medication has not taken effect.

Massage routine

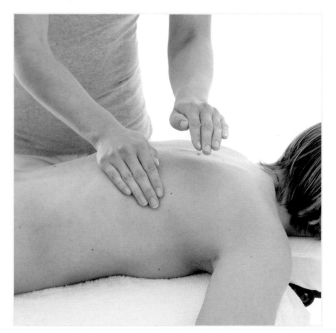

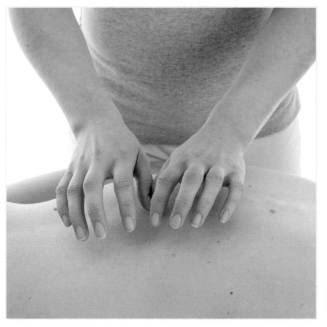

1 With the client lying prone in a comfortable position, apply a cupping stroke over the whole of the back area, avoiding the vertebral column. This is useful between attacks and will promote the release of any build-up of mucus. Be prepared to interrupt the treatment to allow for coughing or the expulsion of congestion.

2 Using tapping techniques, apply friction to the intercostal spaces (between the ribs). This will help to promote lymph flow, stimulate localized cardiovascular flow and relax the muscles, which in turn will ease breathing difficulties.

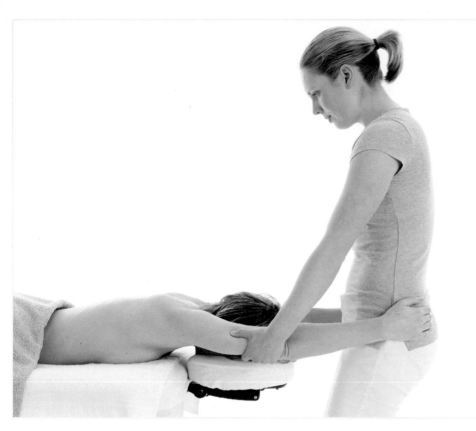

3 Passive stretching will help expand the whole of the respiratory area and encourage easy breathing. Standing upright at the end of the table, hook the client's hands around your lower back and, supporting their upper arms just above the elbows, ask them to take a deep breath in. As they inhale, flex your knees and lean backwards. Maintain the stretch until they exhale and then ease off the traction of the stretch. Keep the support and straighten your knees, ready to repeat.

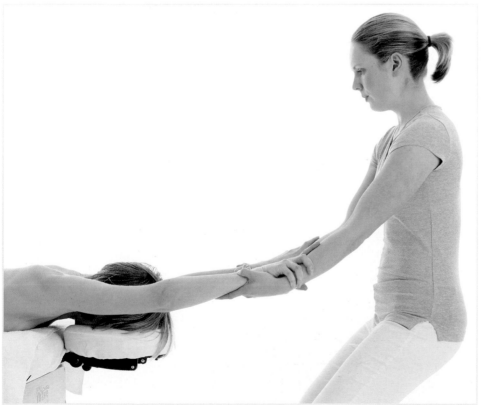

4 In the same position as step 3, slide your supporting hands down the forearms until the client's hands are gripping yours and stretch. This will give a deeper stretch, as you will be able to lean back further, expanding the upper torso more. Before attempting the passive stretch, explain to the client exactly what you are going to do, to avoid any anxiety that may exacerbate their condition.

Menstrual problems and menopause

Many women find that problems associated with both menstruation and menopause, such as period pains, bloating, premenstrual syndrome (PMS), hot flushes and stress, can be helped by massage.

Menstruation is a complicated process and because it is governed by hormones it is associated with all sorts of emotional states. During a woman's child-bearing years, eggs are released from the ovaries every 28 days. If they are fertilized, they attach to the thickened lining of the uterus, but if fertilization does not occur, this lining is not needed and it is expelled via the vagina over a period of three to five days.

A woman will have approximately 500 periods during her lifetime and some women may experience a degree of discomfort during menstruation, such as localized pain or cramps. They may also feel nauseous, fatigued and lack-lustre. Massage can help reduce cramping by relaxing the muscle, help with tiredness by stimulation of the immune system and generally promote a feeling of well-being.

A woman is said to have reached the menopause once she has not had a period for one year. The average age of

natural menopause is 52 years old, although it may take place prematurely in the 40s or much later. Menopause may also be brought forward as a result of invasive treatments such as chemotherapy or radiotherapy and the surgical procedure hysterectomy, in which the uterus is removed.

During the peri-menopausal period various hormonal changes happen: the ovaries gradually reduce hormone production until it stops altogether and the ovaries become scar tissue. These changes can cause unpleasant physical and emotional problems including hot flushes, night sweats, insomnia, weight gain, concentration problems, urinary changes, reduced libido, heart palpitations and headaches.

Massage can reduce the stress and anxiety of this transitional period and help with depression, mood swings, memory and fatigue. The following routine can be used for both menstrual and menopausal problems.

Massage routine

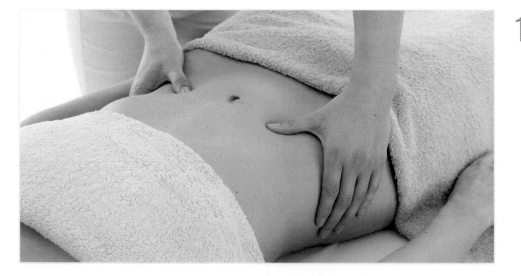

1 Place the pads of the thumbs approximately 7 cm (3 in) either side of the navel. Using your body weight, lean in towards the navel and hold the position for five seconds before releasing. Repeat four to five times.

2 Move the thumbs closer together and using the pads, apply the technique as in Step 1, but reposition after each release downwards in a straight line, from just below the navel until level with the hips. Work back up, finishing with the thumbs about 7 cm (3 in) on either side of the navel.

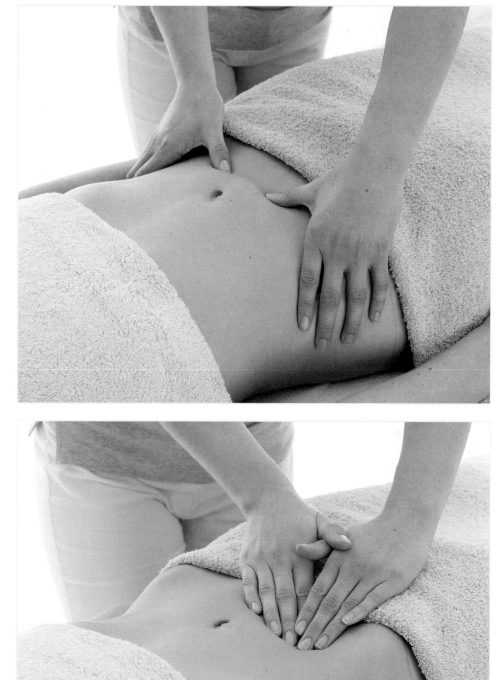

3 With your hands relaxed and close together, place them on the mid-abdominal area level with the navel. Using light strokes, effleurage gently in an arc towards the groin and then return. Make sure that both sides of the abdomen are massaged equally for a balanced treatment. You may wish to substitute an intermittent pressure technique for effleurage. This time the pads of the fingers instead of sliding, stretch the tissues by applying and releasing pressure as you trace an arc towards the groin. This movement is very subtle and you should remain in contact at all times.

Oedema

Oedema, or fluid retention, can occur in any part of the body, but it is common in the hands, arms, legs, ankles and feet, where it causes visible swelling and puffiness. Because oedema is usually a symptom of an underlying condition, any unexplained occurrence, particularly around the ankles, should be checked by a physician.

Housemaid's knee

One of the areas of the body particularly prone to oedema is the knee. This causes what used to be called 'housemaid's knee', in which the sac of fluid in front of the kneecap becomes inflamed and swollen. Housemaids were prone to this condition because kneeling for long periods puts extra pressure on the knee.

Manual lymphatic drainage

Oedema in the upper arms can occur due to hormonal changes, excessive exercising or a disorder that affects the flow of lymph. It can also occur following a masectomy that included removal of the lymph nodes. Build up of such fluids can be treated with massage and manually drained from the area with a specialized technique called manual lymphatic drainage. The application of regular massage strokes will also promote the flow of lymph.

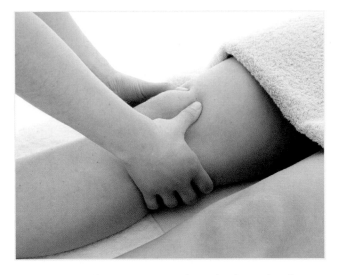

Working on one leg at a time, use the pads of your thumbs to work around the area surrounding the knee joint. Position your thumbs at the top of the area and lean into the area, directing the pressure towards the centre. Hold for three seconds and release before sliding the thumbs to the next postion and repeating the process. You will feel a natural groove around the knee joint. Work around each side until you have reached the area underneath and completed a full circle. Repeat on the other leg. Always check that the pressure is comfortable for the client and if you are only treating the localized area, finish off with some effleurage on the lower limbs and the feet.

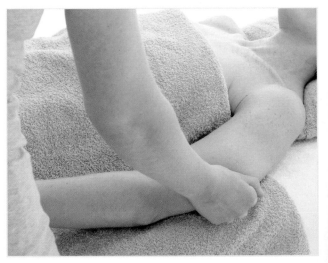

Support the client's arm by resting their forearm on yours, at the same time holding the underside of the elbow. With the working hand, lean into the outside area of the upper arm and using the petrissage squeezing technique, slowly work over the muscle upwards from the elbow to the shoulder. Return using flat-handed effleurage down the outside of the arm, repeating four or five times before moving on to the other arm. Even though only one arm may be affected, there is a need to massage both sides of the body in the same way or the client may feel a disorientation or lack of balance with the overall treatment.

Leg cramps

A cramp is a painful muscle spasm that occurs when a muscle contracts too hard. The most common are stomach cramps and leg cramps. A leg cramp is usually located in the calf muscle and sometimes affects the small muscles in the feet.

Cramp is an acute condition only lasting a short time from seconds up to a few minutes, but it can be excruciatingly painful and can leave the muscle feeling tender for up to 24 hours. Leg cramps tend to occur at night and may disturb sleep. They are more frequent in older people and about four in ten people experience cramps three times a week or more. It may be a sign of arteriosclerosis or hardening of the arteries.

Leg cramps can happen for many reasons, including overexertion of the muscles, dehydration, medications and poor circulation. They may also be the result of the muscle already resting in a shortened position, such as having the knees flexed where further contraction would cause muscle spasm.

Stretching and massage can relieve the condition and soothe muscle discomfort.

Massage routine

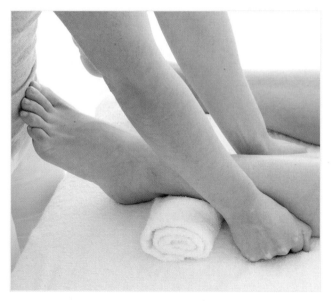

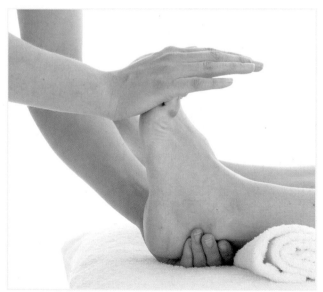

1 Working on the localized area and with fingers of both hands closed, not splayed, cup them around the back of the calf with the tips of the fingers of each hand facing each other along the midline of the muscle. Exert pressure with both hands simultaneously, rolling the muscle by applying the petrissage kneading technique. Release the pressure and repeat, slowly working up the whole muscle affected to reduce muscle tension and spasm.

2 Supporting the ankle with one hand, flex the foot to the point of resistance, pushing the toes and ball of the foot forward using the open palm of the working hand. Reverse the action by pulling back the foot whilst pushing down on the heel with the supporting hand. This passive stretching will help to release and stretch out the muscle, and promote the flow of fresh blood supply to the muscle, slowly reducing the cramping.

Shoulder stiffness

Shoulder symptoms are characterized by restricted movements and pain. The joint capsule and the surrounding muscle may be inflamed, resulting in stiffness and contraction, which in turn affect movement. If the pain is unbearable, the person stops using the joint, giving the condition the name 'frozen shoulder'.

The pain associated with frozen shoulder, or adhesive capsulitis, tends to increase with movement of the affected joint and so there is a tendency to rest the shoulder and worsen the condition by shortening the muscle range. Stiffness is experienced in the run-up to the 'freezing' stage and this can last for long periods. It affects adduction of the arm and rotation of the shoulder, and if not addressed can eventually restrict all shoulder and arm movements.

Massage can help in alleviating the stiffness and preventing the onset of frozen shoulder in the first or acute stage. Other bodywork can also be very effective.

Massage routine

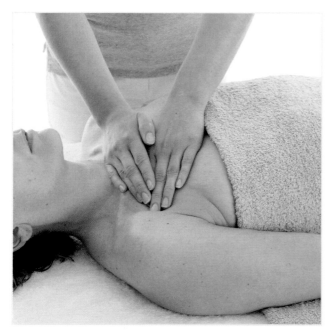

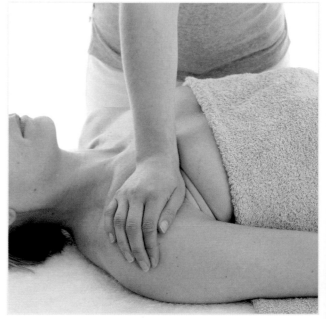

1 Working side-on, place the flat of both hands on the central chest in line with the ribcage. Apply flat-handed effleurage, gliding sideways upwards, moving across the top of the shoulder to its outer edge and return down the outer side of the upper torso to the initial point of contact. Repeat several times as necessary.

2 Place the upper hand on the pectoral muscle furthest away from you. Applying pressure through the heel of the hand, glide across the muscle over the top of the shoulder, returning with reduced pressure. Repeat as necessary.

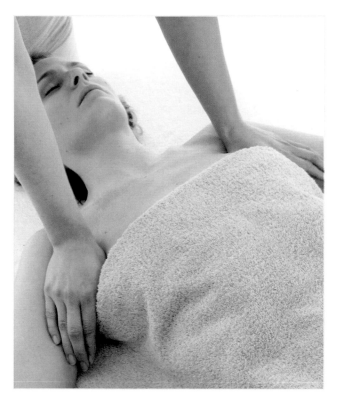

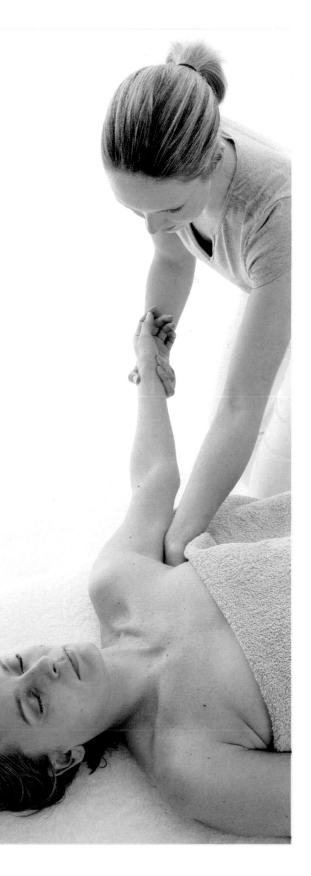

3 Keeping contact, move to the head of the table, lean forward and place both hands at the top of the pectoral muscles, fingers towards the edge of the chest area. Making sure your arms are straight, apply firm pressure with a slight push downwards in order to open up the shoulder area. This is a press and stretch technique so take care not to glide. Repeat as necessary.

4 Passive stretching can also help shoulder stiffness. Working side-on, support the upper arm with both hands, placing one hand on the underside of the shoulder joint. Moving gently, lift the shoulder very slightly. In the same position, slide your other hand down to the wrist for support and pull the arm forwards and outwards until a comfortable point of resistance is reached and release. From the same position, pull the arm outwards and downwards, holding the stretch for as long as is comfortable and release.

Neck strain

The neck is a delicate area, balancing the weight of the head on just seven vertebrae, alongside of which extend vital nerves and blood vessels in a complex structure. Hardly surprising then, that it is prone to strain.

Some neck strains are the result of specific injury such as a car accident, others can be work-related due to poor ergonomics or the need to keep the head in one position for long periods (e.g. dentists). A simple cause can be poor sleeping positions that result in waking up with a neck strain.

In most cases neck strain and the accompanying pain is caused by habitual poor posture or tension. The tension in turn tightens up the muscles in the neck and results in pain that can range from a dull ache to immobility.

Massage routine

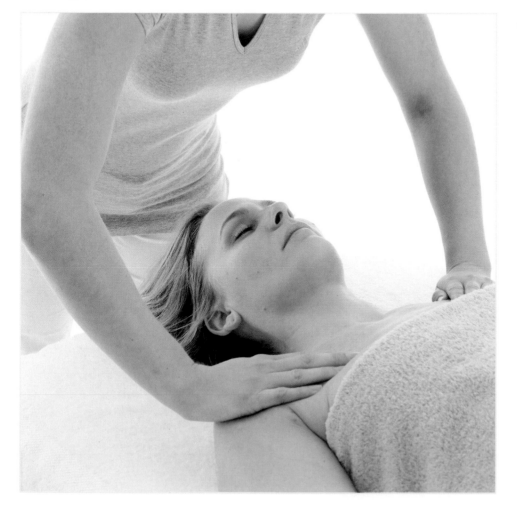

1 Positioning yourself at the top of the table, with the client supine, make contact on the top of each arm and with a flat-handed effleurage stroke warm up the area over the top of the shoulders and base of the neck, scooping your hands underneath the area for the return stroke.

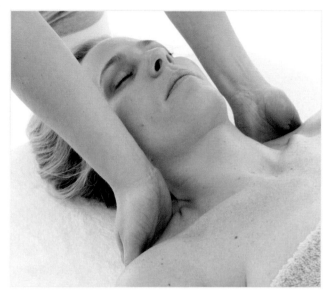

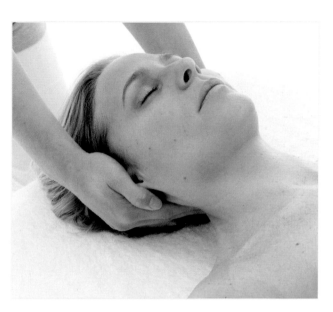

2 With hands in a palm-down position, continue with the effleurage stroke up underneath the neck until they overlap.

3 From the same position, cup your hands under the neck close to the base of the skull and pull them slowly back towards you, at the same time slightly leaning back to facilitate a very gentle neck stretch without the need to lift the head.

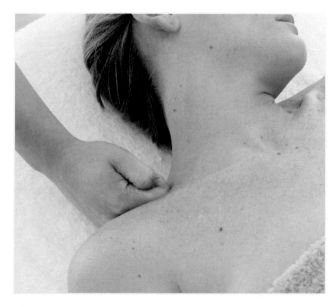

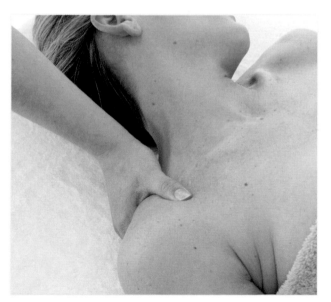

4 Ask the client to move the head sideways away from the side being worked on. Keeping contact with one hand, use the working hand to apply the 'du poing' effleurage stroke (see page 234) gliding outwards with the flat of the fist along the back of the shoulder from the base of the neck to the top of the arm, keeping it flat to the surface. At the end of the stroke, ease off the pressure and return the hand to the base of the neck.

5 With the opened web of the hand, glide down the neck with the palm and fingers making contact on the underside, apply gentle pressure and push outwards towards the top of the arm. Ask the client to turn their head to the opposite side enabling you to work on the other side of the neck.

Massage routine *continued*

6 Place both hands flat down on the shoulders and, using firm pressure, push down, then release in a flowing action, one hand pushing as the other releases. Repeat as necessary.

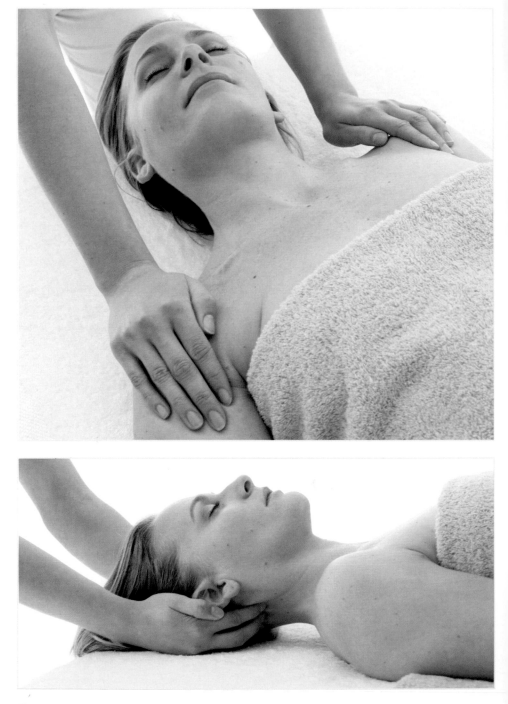

7 Glide the hands upwards, either side of the neck, resting the pads of the fingers on the occipital ridge at the base of the skull. With the pads, apply pressure using a small circular movement, at the same time rotating the fingers. As you are applying this stroke, lean your weight back slightly to action a slight stretch to the neck. Finish off by combing your fingers through the hair, to the top of the skull. Ask the client to turn their head to the opposite side and repeat the technique on the other side of the neck.

Irritable bowel syndrome

IBS, as it is often called, is a chronic disorder of the digestive tract. The digestive and bowel function is impaired, but there is no physical damage visible and no obvious cause.

In the UK one in five people develop IBS at some stage in life, but it more frequently affects teenagers and young adults, and women more often than men. The symptoms are recurring abdominal pain or discomfort, bloating and intermittent diarrhoea, often alternating with constipation. The pain is sometimes described as a spasm or colic and can vary in severity. Symptoms are not constantly present and they can be eased with treatment.

Occasionally the condition can also cause nausea, headaches and fatigue. Although the cause of IBS is not clear, it is generally thought to be related to overactivity in some parts of the digestive tract, resulting in an imbalance. If the muscles that cause food to pass through the tract become overactive or abnormal in any way, the bowel is then irritated. Massage can promote relaxation, which in turn can calm spasms.

Massage routine

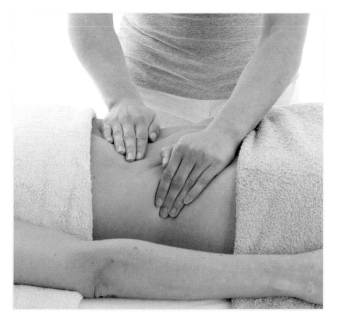

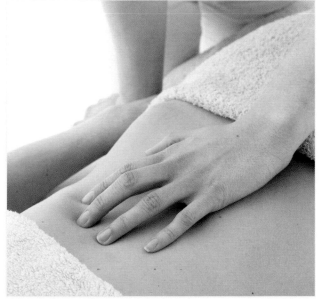

1 Warm the abdominal area with gentle effleurage, position yourself side-on and place your hands on the opposite sides of the abdomen, slightly cupped over the sides of the torso. It is important to apply even pressure through both the palms and the fingers for this technique. Push one hand forward and the other back, simultaneously using the petrissage stroke across the whole of the abdomen from near to far side in one large movement.

2 Place one hand just below the ribcage with the pads of the fingers slightly splayed and facing up the body. Apply a vibrational stroke, using the pads of the fingers to exert pressure and at the same time making minute circular movements with each fingertip simultaneously. This is a very small movement, stimulating the descending colon with the aim of promoting movement along the digestive tract.

Plantar fasciitis

A painful inflammation of the arch tendon of the foot, plantar fasciitis is usually caused by overuse, hence the common name 'policeman's heel'. The pain on the underside of the heel radiates through the foot and is particularly noticeable first thing after waking.

If untreated, plantar fasciitis can lead to a bony growth known as a heel spur, where the tendon attaches to the calcaneus or heel bone. This condition is often associated with runners and dancers, where excessive stretching or landing from heights occur on a regular basis. The most common symptoms are burning, stabbing or aching pains in the heel of the foot. One of the common causes is the presence of very tight calf muscles, which repetitively overstretches the plantar fascia. Massaging the calf muscles may also help with this condition, as will some self-help techniques. When there is a need to relieve pain and discomfort or to stretch out the area at the start of the day, place a tennis ball under the arch of the foot and roll it backwards and forwards over the length of the plantar fascia, from heel to toe. To reduce acute pain use a cold drinks can as a substitute for the tennis ball.

Massage routine

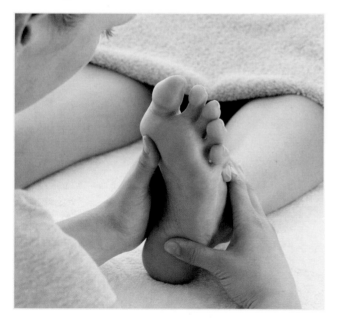

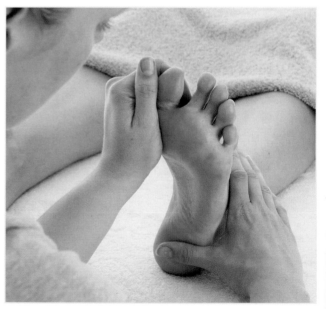

1 Position yourself at the foot of the table and take the foot in both hands, wrapping your fingers around the top of the foot with your thumbs on the sole. Using the whole length of the thumbs, pull them in opposite directions towards the outer edges of the foot, applying deep friction massage across the sole. If the client can tolerate it, continue to the heel of the foot at the insertion to the calcaneus point. Repeat as necessary.

2 Using the heel of the hand, push into the ball of the foot, applying deep pressure and work down towards the heel in a push and release technique. Make sure the pressure is tolerable as any discomfort will cause a tightening up reflex.

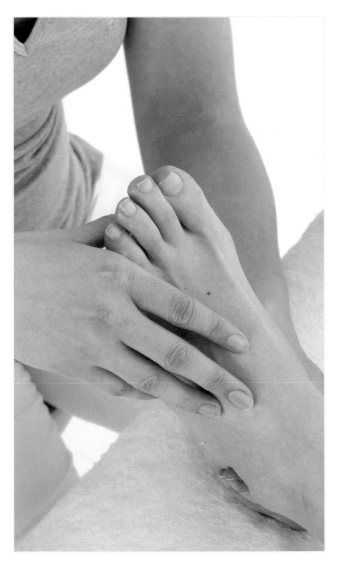

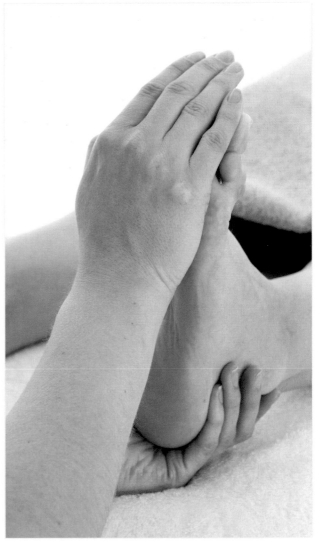

3 Moving to the top of the foot, apply light stroking techniques over the area and finish over the metatarsals. With your fingers placed under the ball of the foot for support, use the thumb to glide outwards, opening up the metatarsal bones.

4 Once the whole foot has been warmed up, some passive stretching will help the condition. With one hand supporting the heel of the foot, use the heel of the working hand placed underneath the toes to push the top of the foot forwards in a dorsiflexion movement. Only push until resistance is felt, hold for five seconds and, using the flats of the fingers hooked over the top of the toes, move the foot back gently to the starting position. Repeat as necessary. Treat the other foot.

Deep vein thrombosis

DVT or deep vein thrombosis, a condition linked with sitting inactively for long periods of time such as in a plane or car, is well publicized and airlines have taken responsibility to educate their passengers on preventative measures.

Known commonly as 'economy class syndrome', DVT is the formation of a blood clot, usually in the calf area, which causes swelling and pain. If this clot were to move and travel around the body it could end up lodged in the lung and be potentially fatal.

Veins do not have a muscular wall to pump blood back to the heart, but rely on a system of valves and the assistance of the muscles of the calf and lower leg to pump the blood onwards. If there is no muscle activity, the blood flow slows down and a clot may form.

During a long flight there are some preventative measures that will help reduce the risk of DVT: keep hydrated by drinking water, do not cross the legs – this puts pressure on the blood vessels at the back of the legs, make sure socks and shoes are not constrictive, and move regularly if possible. Anyone who has varicose veins or who has had recent injury or surgery to the legs should wear special support hose during the flight.

Massage can manually assist the blood flow through the deep veins and their valves in the legs onwards towards the heart, which is normally done through regular movement and pressure.

If a client is prone to DVT, a professional massage after a flight is advisable to stimulate venous flow. The therapist should apply the strokes described here plus further friction work.

This simple routine can also be self-applied through the clothes during a flight, whilst in a seated position. A variation for self-massage during a flight is to use an inflatable travelling neck pillow; place each foot either side of the 'u' shape and simply press down alternately, letting the air pump the feet upwards and downwards.

Massage routine

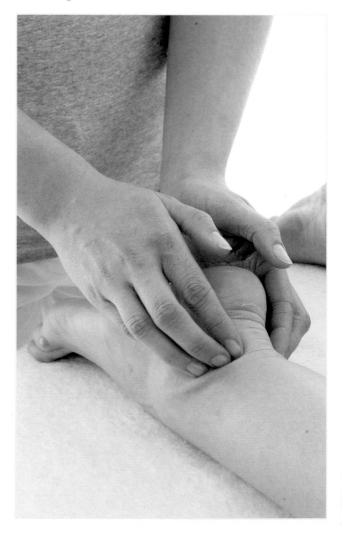

1 With the client prone, apply both hands to one leg at a time. Place the pads of your fingers either side of the foot between the ankle and the heel. Working in a small circular movement, apply intermittent pressure as though manually pumping the area. Repeat on the other leg.

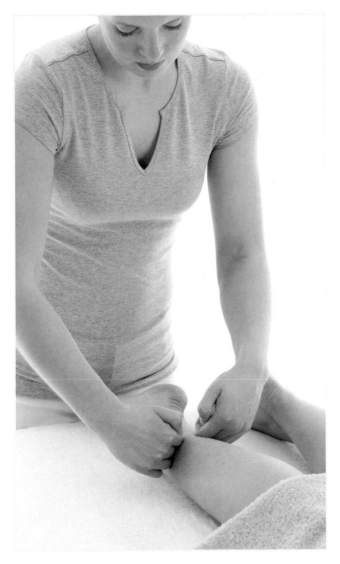

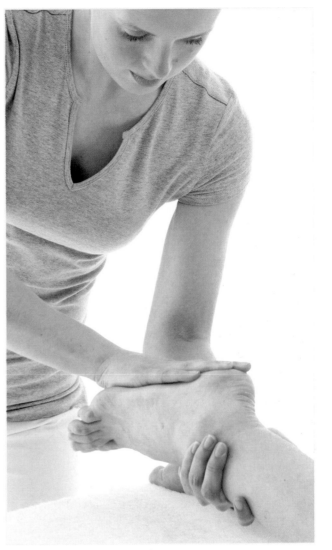

2 Using the knuckling stroke, work both hands upwards from the ankle towards the knee area and return, the pressure always on the upward stroke. Apply the stroke in a straight or circular movement over the sides or back of the calves, avoiding any varicose veins. Repeat several times before moving to the other leg.

3 Supporting the ankle with one hand, lift the foot slightly off the table, place the palm of the working hand on the sole of the foot and alternatively apply pressure to the heel and then the toe in a pumping action, moving the foot forwards and backwards to encourage venous flow. Repeat on the other leg.

Repetitive strain injury

Repetitive strain injury or RSI is a real health problem in the workplace. An umbrella term covering non-specific arm pain, regional pain disorders and carpal tunnel syndrome, it is caused by mechanical irritation, a result of constantly repeating similar physical movements and is a self-inflicted injury relating to poor biomechanics.

Often associated with using a keyboard, any prolonged static load on muscles or repetitive action can cause RSI. It is a common condition in musicians, check-out operators, assembly-line workers and cleaners. Even housework or a hobby can result in RSI if poor posture, technique or the wrong equipment is employed.

Symptoms are progressive and initially include swelling, redness and a reduction in range of movement. As the condition progresses, coldness, tingling or numbness may occur and the pain becomes more persistent, even after rest periods. Chronic RSI results in deterioration of the joints and arthritis and some conditions, such as carpal tunnel syndrome, where the nerves passing between the arm and hand through the wrist are compressed by inflamed tendon sheaths, may require surgery.

Massage, together with re-education of work habits and improved ergonomics, will help prevent the onset of RSI or help manage the condition. Massage of the forearms, pectoralis major and minor and the neck areas will help range of movement. Building up the posterior forearm muscles with exercise will also benefit the condition.

Massage routine

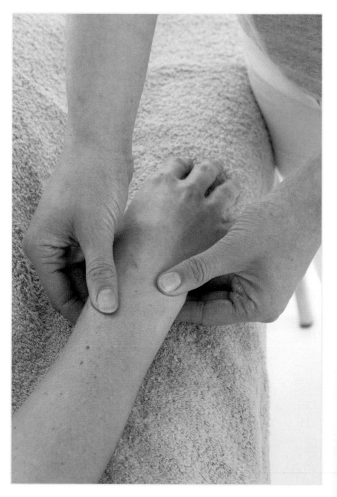

1 With the arm palm down, place the pads of your thumbs on the top of the wrist, supporting it with your fingers. Apply pressure, working in circular movements over the wrist area, thumbs rotating in opposite directions.

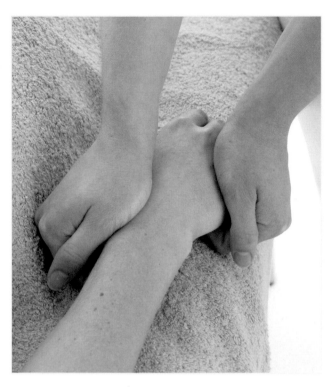

2 Placing the heels of both hands centrally on the top of the hand, glide off in opposite directions to the end of the area, applying pressure and stretching out the area.

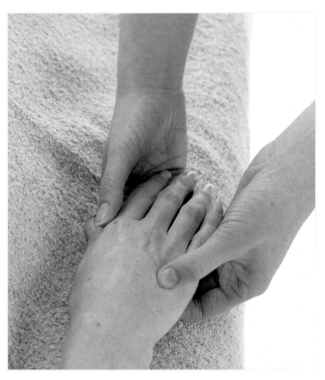

3 With one hand supporting your client's hand, place the thumb pad of your working hand between the third and fourth fingers, just above the web and glide up towards the wrist, applying pressure. Move to the top of the web between the second and third fingers and repeat applying pressure through the groove between the knuckles up towards the wrist. Repeat, moving along the hand until all four areas have been massaged.

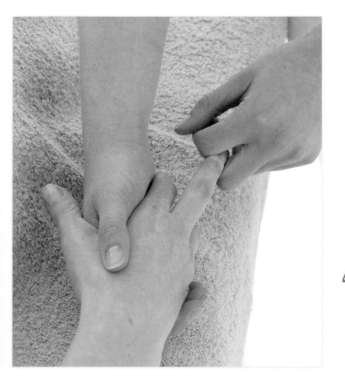

4 Placing the flat of your hand under your client's hand for support, in a handshake clasp, take the little finger at the base between your thumb and index finger and gently slide down the length of the finger, stretching and slightly twisting the digit before pulling off at the tip. Move along the hand to work each finger and the thumb before repeating the sequence on the other hand.

Poor circulation

Poor circulation usually affects the extremities of the body – the fingers, toes, ears and nose – and can be caused by a variety of conditions that restrict the blood flow through the blood vessels in these parts.

One of the more serious conditions is Raynaud's syndrome, in which the small arteries of the hands and feet go into periodic spasms and constrict. Commonly these episodes follow exposure to cold or emotional stress and the condition can lead to permanent nerve damage and even tissue destruction. The feet in particular will be very cold, pale and sometimes feel numb.

Massage will promote circulation, the pressure used being dependent on the tolerance of the client. The use of heat and ice packs is contraindicated for Raynaud's and you should ensure that the feet are well covered when not being worked on. You may also find it more soothing to use powder or wax instead of oil for this particular routine.

Massage routine

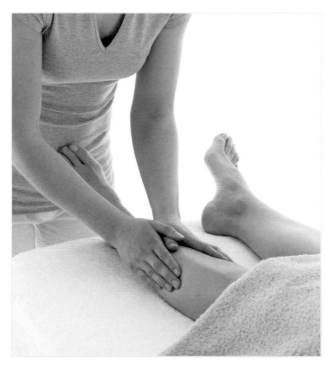

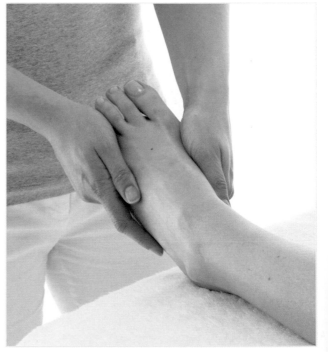

1 Place the flat of your hands on the top of the foot with one thumb on top of the other. Use light pressure and as you breathe out, work up the front of the foot towards the lower leg. Glide back down either side of the foot, leaning backwards slightly to add a stretch to the stroke. Repeat three to five times.

2 Rest your thumbs and heels of hand on the top of the foot with your fingers wrapped around the sides of the foot you are working on. Draw your thumbs across the foot in opposite directions, squeezing the foot firmly and bringing them down to join the rest of your hand in a movement that stretches and opens up the area.

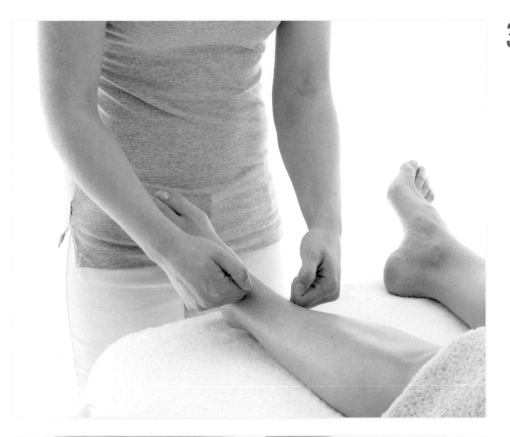

3 Make your hands into loose fists and apply the knuckling stroke, circling all over the top and sides of the foot. Repeat several times before moving to the other foot to repeat the sequence.

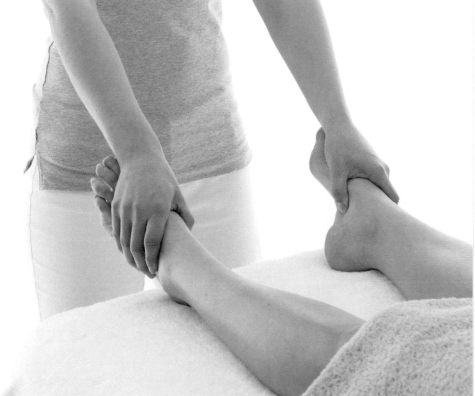

4 To finish, place each hand over the corresponding foot, palm down with thumb pads on the instep and finger pads on the outer edge of the client's feet and apply pressure, holding for a few seconds before releasing. This routine can be used alone or as a continuation of a leg massage.

Trigeminal neuralgia

Often triggered by everyday activities such as eating, talking or even brushing the teeth, trigeminal neuralgia is characterized by episodes of intense, stabbing pains in the face, usually on one side only.

Sometimes known as cranial nerve V, the trigeminal nerve has three branches that carry sensations from various parts of the face: ophthalmic – eye nasal capacity, forehead upper eyelid and eyebrow; maxillary – lower eyelid, upper lip, gums, teeth, cheek nose and some parts of the pharynx; mandibular – lower gums, teeth, lower lip, palate and part of the tongue. The trigeminal nerve is the one locally anaesthetized by the dentist when carrying out work.

The neuralgia or pain associated with any one branch of this nerve can be excruciating, but little is known about why it occurs. The pain can vary greatly in duration and only light strokes should be administered, avoiding any area that elicits pain.

Massage routine

Trigeminal neuralgia of the first branch most commonly affects the forehead and eyes, and the following simple routine may help with pain relief.

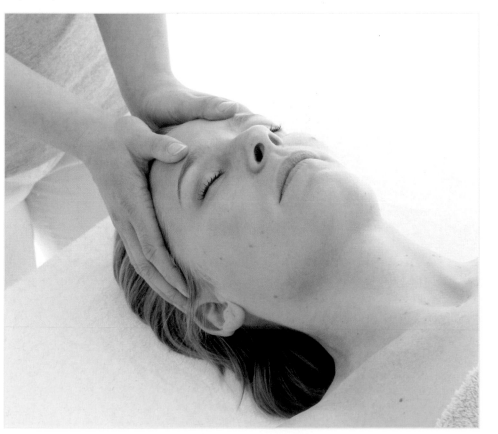

1 Make contact, resting the pads of the thumbs next to each other on the forehead. Glide the flat of each thumb outwards towards the edge of the area, lift off and return slowly, working over the whole area from the hairline to the brow line.

2 Taking great care and having made sure the client has removed contact lenses, glide the thumb pads across the eyelids from the corner of the eye to the outer edge and return. If the pain is too great, action the stroke but do not make contact.

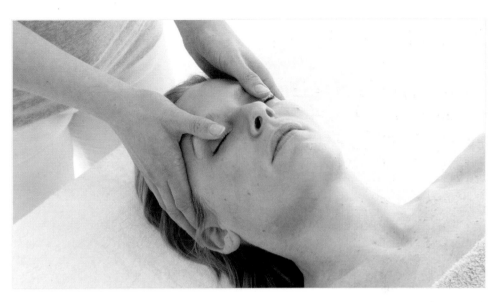

3 Place the index and middle finger pads of each hand on the corresponding temples, apply slight pressure, hold for a few seconds and release.

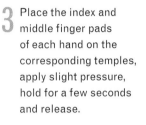

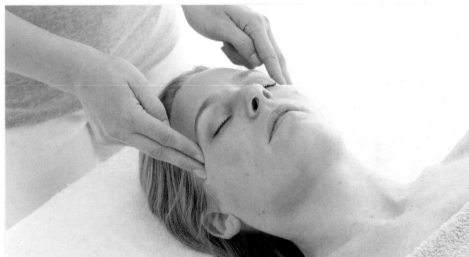

4 Repeat as many times as required and finish off by taking very small strands of hair from around the hairline between the thumb and finger pads and use both hands alternately to very lightly pull upwards and off.

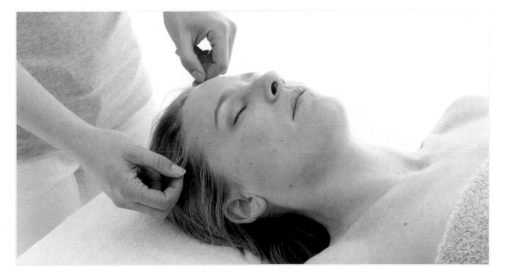

Eye strain

With the increased use of computers, electronic media and the brightness of halogen lighting, eye strain has become a common complaint, particularly at the end of a working day.

Sensations to and from the eyes are carried through two cranial nerves: CNII the optic nerve and CNIII the oculomotor, which controls four of the six eye muscles that allow the eyeball to move. The effects of strain on these nerves and muscles can cause blurred vision, headaches and even migraines.

A simple massage routine can be applied by the therapist or used with reversed hand positions as a self-massage routine whilst in a seated position.

Massage routine

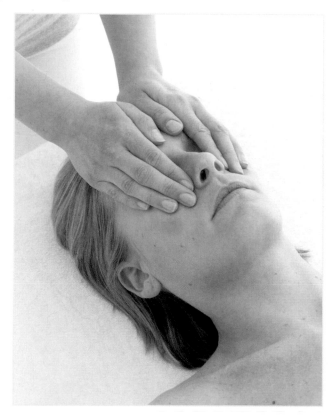

1 Positioned at the top of the table, place your hands at the top of the forehead with the palm of each hand over the corresponding eye, finger pads resting on the top of the cheekbones. Slowly apply a little pressure over the closed eyelids and hold for a few seconds before releasing.

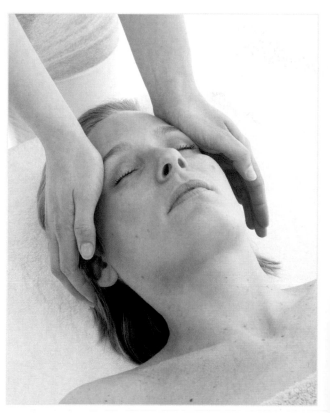

2 Position the heel of each hand on the corresponding eyebrow and glide outwards from the inner end of the brow to the side of the head an pull off, smoothing the entire length of the eyebrow, repeating as necessary.

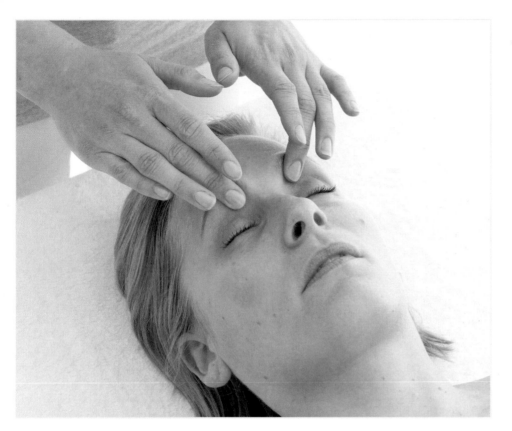

3 Returning to the position at the inner end of the eyebrow, place the pad of each thumb or middle finger, whichever is more comfortable, under the edge of the brow bone. Apply light pressure and hold for a few seconds before releasing, repeating as necessary.

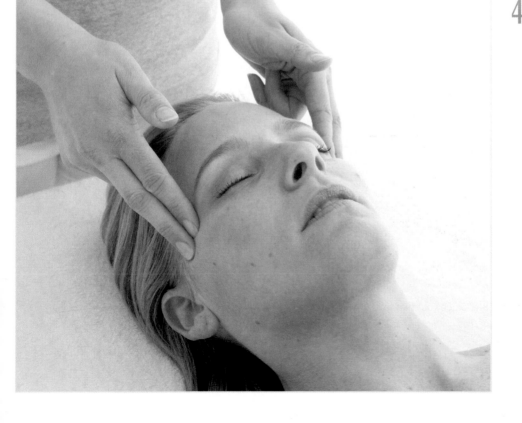

4 To finish, place the pads of the middle two fingers on the corresponding temples and rotate anti-clockwise, applying a little pressure at the same time (clockwise for self-massage routine).

Shin splints

Shin splints, or periostitis, refers to pain felt at the front of the lower leg. The membrane lining the tibia, known as the periosteum, becomes inflamed and friction from the leg muscles rubbing against this causes pain along the shin.

A particular condition affecting runners, shin splints often disappear after a period of rest, only to return when running commences. Massage can promote relaxation of the muscles in the lower leg, which will reduce the friction and heat against the periosteum and help the healing process.

Massage routine

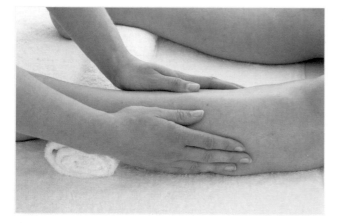

1 Working on one leg at a time, position both hands just above the ankle and apply flat-handed effleurage upwards to just below the knee, returning down the outsides of the leg, covering as much area as possible. Keep the pressure light and at a level tolerable to the client. Repeat as necessary.

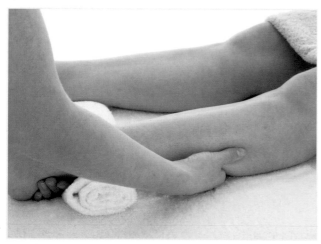

2 Position the hand palm upwards underneath the back of the shin and with the pad of the thumb glide up the posterior muscles, applying firm pressure and avoiding the attachment area.

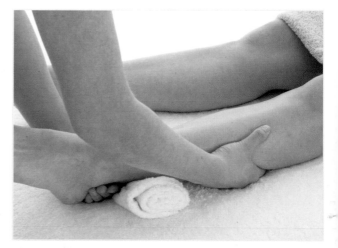

3 Position the hand on the lower part of the shin and with the thumb pad work in short strokes across the muscle, applying cross-friction massage in order to stretch out the fascia, slowly working up the shin, avoiding the actual bone. Finish off with effleurage as in Step 1 to soothe the area.

Golfer's elbow

As the name suggests, this is a condition common in people who play golf. More formally known as lateral epicondylitis, the causes are the same as for tennis elbow but this time relating to the upper rather than lower arm.

The first symptoms of golfer's elbow are pain in the wrist joint when the elbow is extended whilst facing upwards, due to the inflammation of the extensors of the arm. Whilst playing golf, a dull ache tends to occur between the elbow and the shoulder area. The inflammation occurs when an action requires forceful flexion of the wrist or the joints of the shoulder girdle.

Massage routine

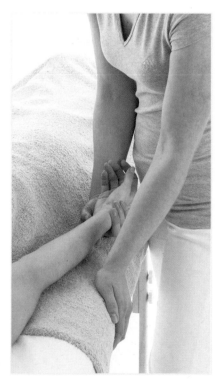 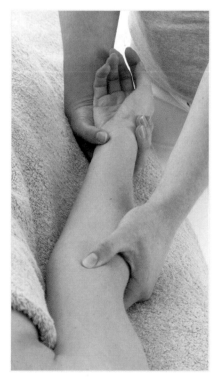 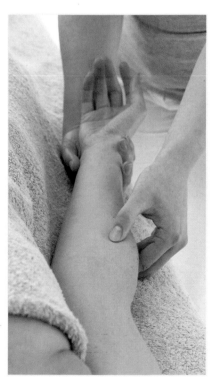

1 With the arm placed palm and forearm upwards, support the wrist with one hand, making sure that the elbow is well supported on the table.

2 Place the pad of the thumb of the working hand on the inside of the elbow and, applying pressure through the thumb, work around the area in small rotations.

3 Keeping the same position, use the tip of the thumb to apply cross friction across the inside of the elbow, by applying pressure whilst moving the thumb backwards and forwards in short dynamic strokes. If the condition is tender, adjust the pressure accordingly.

Pre- and post-sports

Sports and athletics have recognized the benefits of massage and bodywork since the ancient Greek and Roman times, as it was thought to bring athletes to the peak of their performance.

There is clear evidence that massage played a significant role in Ancient Greece at the time of the early Olympic Games, and its use is documented as far back as 25 BC by the likes of Hippocrates, Plato and Galen.

Although massage at sporting events took a back seat again when the original Greek games were terminated in AD393, it was put firmly back on the map by a Finnish runner called Paavo Nurmi in the 20th century. Nurmi brought his own personal massage therapist to the 1924 Olympics in Paris and, after winning five gold medals, claimed that his training programme included special massage treatments. The rest, as they say, is history.

These days, athletes and sporting teams, both amateur and professional, usually travel with a massage therapist as part of their entourage. Treatments can be adapted to all variety of sports and is used pre-, between- and post-event alongside preventative and injury management. Pre-event massage should be carried out the day before, warming up the muscles and only using effleurage and light-pressured petrissage. Post-event massage will speed up the process of expelling waste products such as lactic acid that will have built up in the muscles as a result of vigorous exercise.

Promoting venous flow to tired muscles and replenishing oxygen and nutrients will help speed up the recovery process. However, it is advisable to wait an hour after the event has finished before massaging to achieve maximum benefit.

Pre-event massage routine for back

1 With one hand placed on top of the other in reinforced massage position, make contact in the centre of the back and lean your body weight inwards. Hold for about five to ten seconds and release.

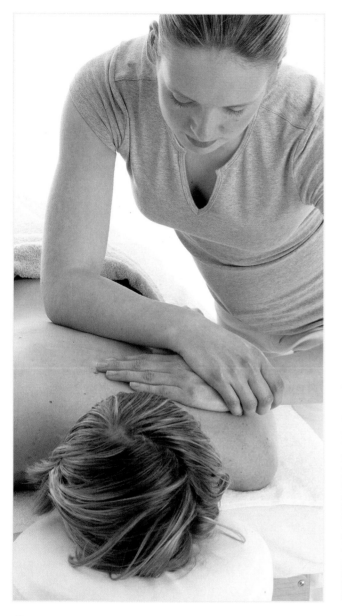

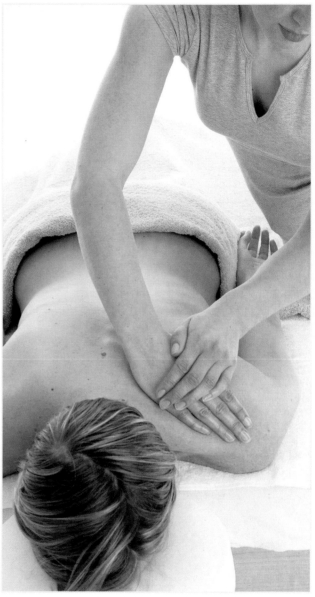

2 Using the flat of your forearm, work at right angles to your upper arm, the opposite hand on top just above the wrist for support. Apply pressure through the arm, guided by the supporting hand and effleurage in a large sweeping arc over one side of the back area.

3 Straighten the arm and pull off slowly in order to repeat the motion on the other side of the back by changing arms. This negates the need to change your working position around the table and is useful if you are applying the massage in the seated postion.

Post-event massage routine for legs

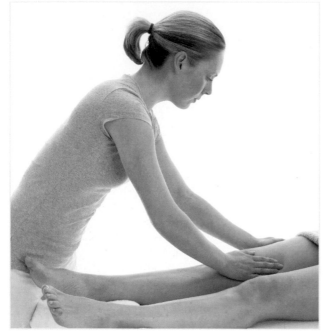

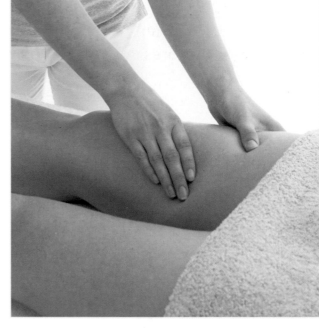

1 Positioning yourself in line with the ankle, apply flat-handed effleurage from the ankle to the knee. Lift off pressure at the knee joint and continue up the thigh. Keep the pressure light and flowing.

2 With an opened web of the hand, fingers and thumbs to one side in a V formation, place one hand on top of the leg just above the ankle, with the other slightly lower on the leg, following behind. Glide up the leg to just below the knee joint, one after the other, returning down the sides of the limb using the flats of the hands. Keeping the hands in the same position start above the knee joint and glide up the thigh as far as is discreet and comfortable, returning down the sides of the thigh, using the flats of the hands.

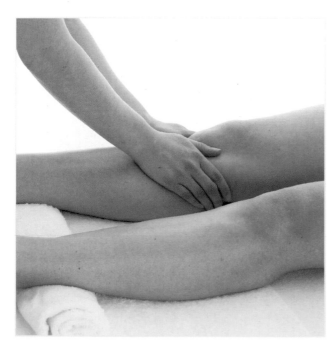

3 As with massage for oedema, work around the knee joint, hooking the fingers either side of the area for support. Using the pads of the thumbs, apply pressure to the natural groove surrounding the joint, using the press and release technique. Work in two arcs either side of the knee from the top to the bottom.

Back pain

The back is a vulnerable area as it is the main support structure of the body and stores large amounts of tension and stress. As a therapist it will be the most common area you will be asked to massage and is also the largest single area you will treat. You may find that some clients will only require the back area to be worked on over shorter, more frequent visits.

Upper back pain refers to pain in the area above the lumbar sacral area, known as the thoracic vertebral area, whereas lower back pain describes pain or tenderness in the lumbar spine. Lower back pain has many symptoms and is usually the result of chronic overuse of the lumbar sacral area. The strain on this area varies when the body assumes different positions; for example, standing creates four times more strain on the lower back than lying on the back with the legs extended.

When a back is in spasm you cannot apply any deep strokes until the whole area has been warmed up and the muscles relaxed; therefore, prior to a heavier stroking action a very light-pressured criss-cross effleurage is used.

Massage routine

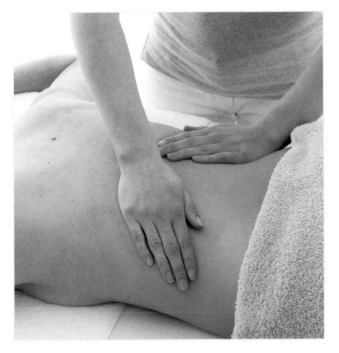

1 Working side-on, place your hands on opposite sides of the lower back area either side of the spine and apply the effleurage stroke, gliding your hands across the back in opposite directions.

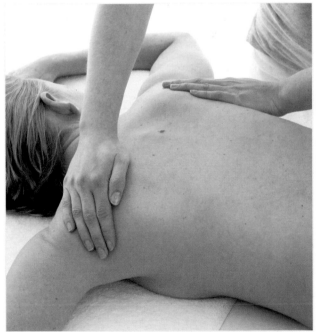

2 Continue working up the back area to the top and then repeat back down to where you started. Keep your rhythm slow, taking around five seconds to glide from one side of the torso to the other.

Massage routine *continued*

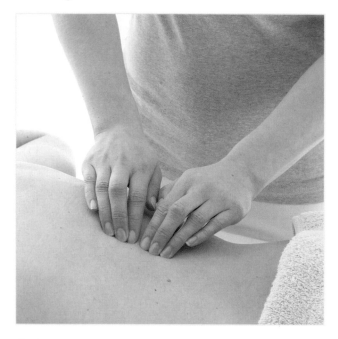

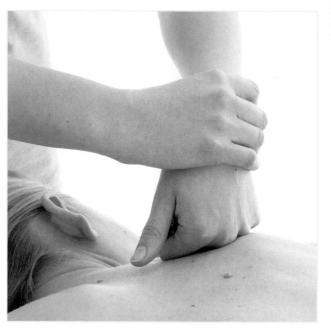

3 Once the muscles are warmed up and relaxed, apply some of the suggested petrissage and friction stokes where required. The following three stokes for back work are versions of effleurage or 'caresse du poing'.

The massaging hand is made into a fist with the fingers straight, resting on the heel of the hand. Place the other hand around the wrist and use to guide the stroke over the lumbar area, applying pressure with the flats on the fingers.

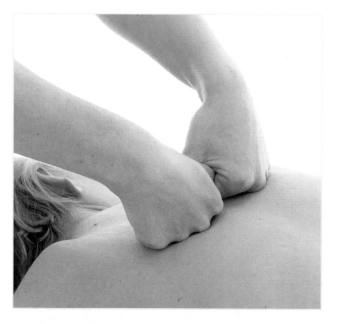

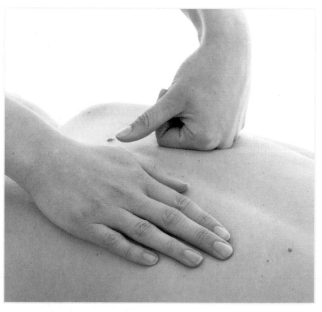

For two handed 'du poing' effleurage, place the thumb of one fist between the thumb and finger of the other for support and apply the stroke so that each fist is either side of the spine. Glide over the lumbar fascia area.

Apply deep pressure to the lumbar muscles with one handed 'du poing' effleurage, using the resting hand to stretch out the lumbar fascia at the same time.

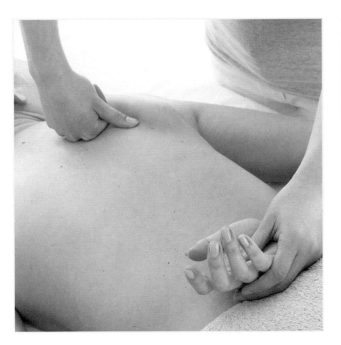

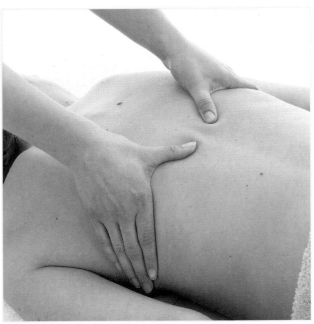

Gently lift the client's arm, resting the hand and wrist on the lower back in order to raise the scapula. With thumb, effluerage along the medial border of the scapula before replacing the arm on the table.

Places the pads of the thumbs either side of the spine, the rest of the hand pointing to the outer edge of the torso for stability, and slowly glide down the lumber area from the top of the scapula to the sacrum. Lift off and repeat as required.

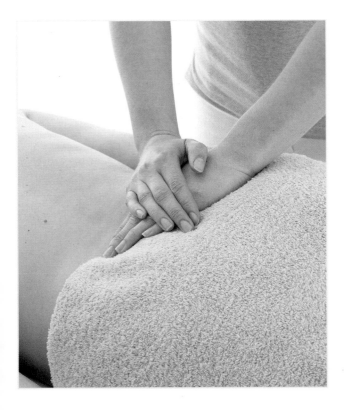

4 Finish off with gentle effleurage over the whole of the lower and upper back areas, resting the hands one on top of the other over the sacrum to finish. Finally, some passive stretching through the arms will open up the whole of the upper back area and reduce strain on the lower area.

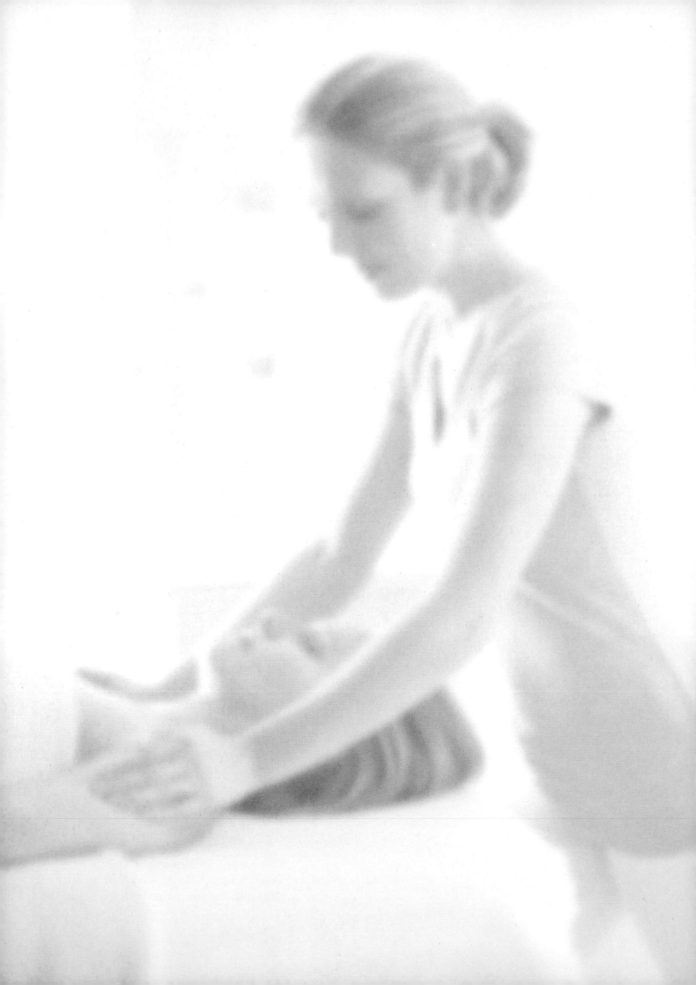

Setting up a massage practice

There are a variety of reasons why people choose to set up their own massage practice. When setting up your own practice you have to ask yourself what you want to get out of it and how you want it to fit in with the rest of your life and build your business around that framework. In this chapter we look at all the aspects of setting up a practice that you will need to consider.

Basic business planning

Many massage therapists love what they do, have great skills but have poor business acumen. Whether you are doing it alone or with a partner, your massage practice is a business and you need to run it efficiently to survive.

As well as performing the massage itself, you will need to handle the appointment bookings, purchase supplies and deal with the financial side of the practice. All this will require a level of organization.

First, you need to give thought to the direction you want your practice to take, identify your expectations and make a vision statement to work towards that will motivate and excite you. Once your vision of the future is clear, move on to writing your mission statement, sometimes called a statement of purpose. Keep it short, read it often and make sure it is flexible so you can revise it as needed.

Being successful relies on having a detailed business plan and following it. Basic planning will enable you to work out where and when you want to work, the marketing mix you will need, priorities, financial guidance and give you the information to apply for a loan or overdraft facility if needed.

Ten primary elements that are needed to develop your business plan are:

1 Your mission statement.
2 The formation of the business. The first important decision to be made is whether you wish to trade alone, in a partnership or as a limited company. There are advantages and disadvantages to each of these options and your local tax office or accountant can give you advice and literature to read to enable you to make an informed decision.
3 An outline of your market, obtained through identifying potential clients and where they are.
4 Details of the services and products you will offer and their unique selling points.
5 A price list and explanation behind the figures.
6 A marketing plan.
7 Analysis of the competition.
8 An identification of your strengths and weaknesses, threats and opportunities (SWOT).
9 Financial considerations.
10 Monitoring the progress of the business.

QUESTIONS TO CONSIDER WHEN SETTING UP A PRACTICE

- Do you want to work full time?
- Do you want to work part time, supplementing another income?
- Do you see this as a career for retirement?
- Are flexible hours and more free time important?
- How do you feel about working for yourself?
- Do you expect personal satisfaction?
- Are you expecting the opportunity to travel and work?
- Do you want to work in sports and with athletes?
- Do you want to work in health care?

What is a mission statement?

A mission statement can be as short as one sentence that summarizes your work ethic and what you aim to provide. This can then be underpinned by a set of values and performance standards.

As a massage therapist your philosophy could be "To offer a safe, professional and relaxed environment to promote better health and lifestyle." An example mission statement could be "To provide massage and integrated bodywork treatments to enhance the physical quality of life and nurture the well-being of the receiver."

Anything that you do in your new business can then be mapped to your mission statement to ensure you are achieving your primary goal.

Business plan Once you have formalized your business plan, revisit it regularly, update where necessary and check that you are achieving your aims and aspirations.

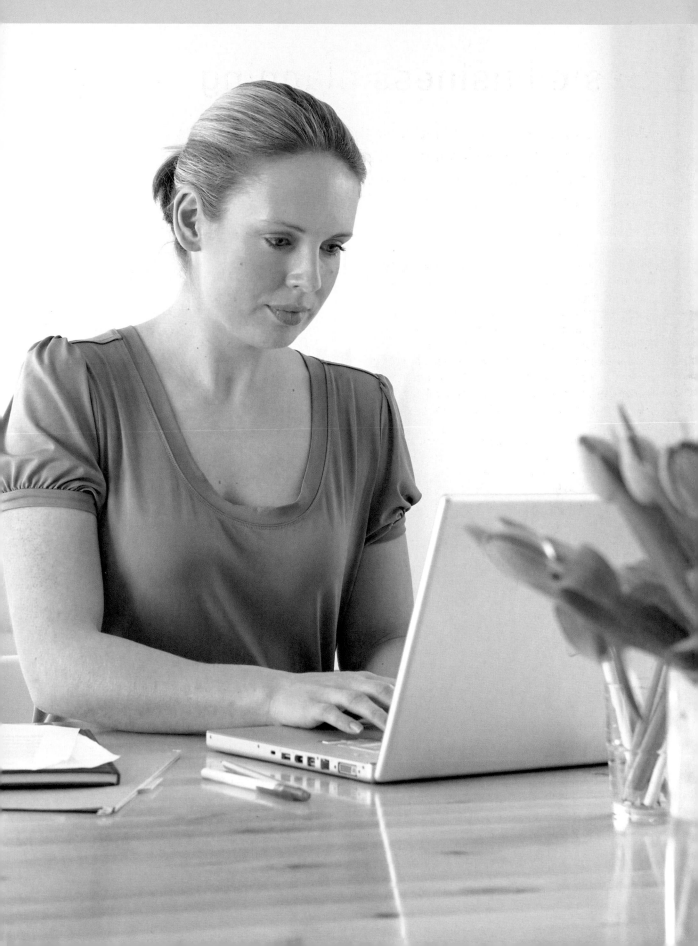

Keeping records

In any type of health practice the keeping of clients' records is important. This has been touched on in a previous chapter, but what are the principles and legal requirements involved?

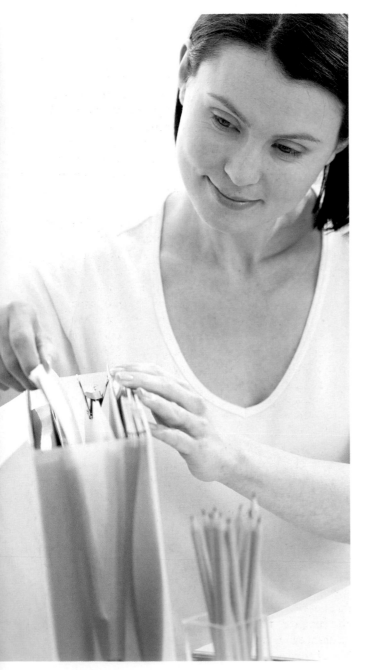

It is imperative that case histories are taken and filed carefully. They must be seen to exist and may need to be produced in the event of legal action. There should therefore be no ambiguous entries or alterations and, if hand written, they should be legible. It can very easy to treat a 'drop in' client without following any formalities, but this is unprofessional and could have consequences, so do not let it happen.

Clients' records should be kept securely. If on paper they should be filed in a locked cabinet; if stored electronically on a computer, they should be protected with a password. Keep a back-up copy in a separate place in case of floods or fire. Current records dating back to the last three years should be kept to hand and older ones archived. Insurance companies often require them to be kept for nine years after the last appointment. Check the terms and conditions of your policy to ensure you comply with any specific requirements. When they are ready to be disposed of, shred or burn the records to ensure confidentiality.

If the client transfers to another therapist who would like to review their notes, obtain permission from the client before handing them over. If you decide to retire or sell your practice, you must make sure that all your clients are informed of the change and given the name of the new therapist. As before, obtain consent to transfer the records on to another. This can be in the form of a simple letter stating that if the client does not register an objection by a certain date you have their permission to hand over the records in your possession.

Where records are kept on computer, you must ensure that you comply with any data protection laws. In the UK you need to register as a keeper under the Data Protection Act 1984 and comply with their rulings.

Clients' records Make sure that all records are kept orderly and accessible. Update a client's record after every visit before storing securely for future reference.

Location and insurance

There are a variety of location options open to the newly trained massage therapist setting up in business. Whether you decide to work with others at a health centre, from a treatment room in your home or indeed as a mobile therapist, there will be regulation and insurance matters you need to deal with.

Having drawn up a business plan and made your financial forecasts you may feel that the risks involved in opening your own venue before you have built up a client base are a little daunting. Alternative ways forward are to work from an established local centre or a treatment room within your own home.

Rules and regulations

Once you have built up a reasonable number of regular weekly clients, you might decide to start researching a venue for your own clinic. If you intend to have your own premises you need to decide whether they will be rented or owned. You will also need to find out about the local regulations and check whether you need to apply for a change of use, for example, if they are not already designated suitable for clinic use. If you take on a lease, will you be committed for a specific length of time and if so, are you allowed to sub-let under the terms of the lease if you need to vacate early?

Other regulations to be considered are the prevailing licence requirements. In the UK there are 17 laws covering health and safety, equipment, products and the consumer, which need to be adhered to. These will apply whether working from home or from other locations.

If working from home you will need to ensure that your household insurers are aware of your business. This may incur an increase in premium.

Similarly you may need to consider tax implications. In the UK, for example, you may be liable for capital gains tax when you sell your house if you have used part of it exclusively for business use.

Professional insurance and registration

Although there may be no statutory requirement to hold insurance as a complementary therapy practitioner in your region, there is definitely an ethical requirement. Your clients will also have more confidence in your professionalism when they see you are fully insured to treat them. In today's litigious climate you need to ensure that you and your clients are adequately protected for professional indemnity and malpractice purposes as well as public liability. Whether you massage only one client a week or one every hour, insurance should be in place and in some cases it is not just desirable, but also a requirement for jobs in the profession.

- **Professional indemnity and malpractice**: This type of insurance covers your actual treatment practices and so you need to check that all the disciplines you carry out in your massage sessions are covered under the policy. You should notify your insurers of any changes, for example, a new qualification or if your client base changes – some insurance companies require a higher premium if a large percentage of your clients are professional sportspeople or dancers.
- **Public liability**: This type of insurance covers accidents that may happen off the massage table, for example, a client slipping on a wet floor or oil spillage on clothing.

Whether you work from home or a clinic, you will still need to have both types of insurance cover. You can also obtain insurance that will cover you whilst you are a student; this can be upgraded once you qualify.

The minimum recommended cover may sound like a very large sum but you should remember that it would need to cover the high costs of legal fees if a case was brought against you that has to be fought in the courts. Even if you have not acted improperly, you will have to spend money to prove the fact, so insurance gives you that peace of mind. If a case was brought against you and compensation awarded to the third party, without insurance in place an enforcement could result in the loss of your personal assets.

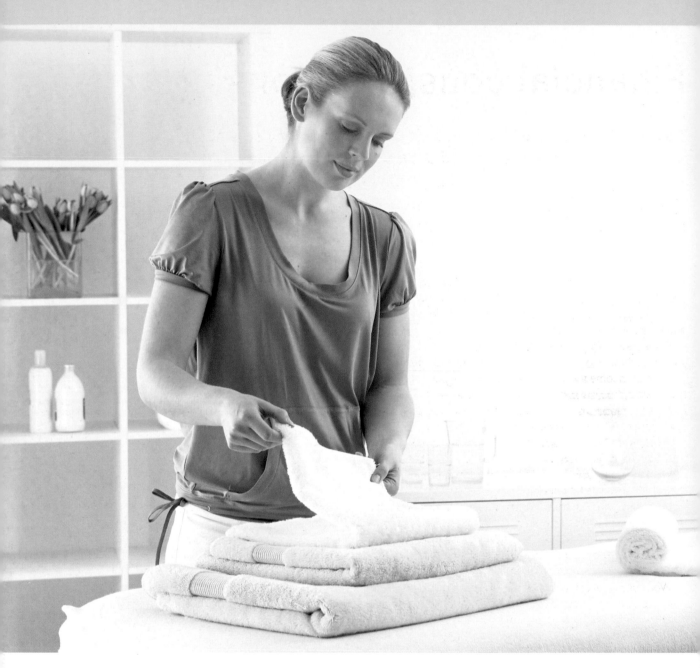

Other types of insurance that you may need to consider are income protection, which will provide you with funds if you are unable to work through illness or injury and help meet rent or mortgage payments. You will also need car insurance for business use for travelling to and from clients and cover for your massage table and accessories in transit. Finally, do not forget to take out contents insurance, covering the tools of your trade, office equipment and loss of records whether at home or in a business property, and building insurance if you run your own clinic building. In the long term you may also wish to consider personal life and health insurance.

Equipment You will require insurance to cover your equipment, as well as the actual treatment, premises and the public while they are in your care.

Massage associations and bodies often run insurance schemes for their members at competitive rates. Their packages are designed to cover all the possible elements required by a massage therapist and they are in a position to offer very good advice. Where an unusal massage discipline is practised, such as equine massage, a specific insurance policy may be needed.

Financial considerations

Your start-up costs will vary greatly depending on the size of the practice, where it is located and the equipment needed. A single-therapist practice, working from home, will require much less capital outlay than a town centre purpose-built practice catering for a range of therapists.

Draw up a realistic list of the money you will need to start your business and what you have available. This will help you to make decisions on where you operate from and whether you take on a partner or partners.

Set a budget forecast for the first five years. This should include expected outgoings and income, the amount of income you need to cover your expenses, a break-even analysis and cash flow projections. If this sounds too complicated, there are simple computer spreadsheets that will calculate the projections for you.

Working to a budget forecast will keep you informed if the business is on track or not and enable you to take remedial action if it is not. It is a good way of monitoring the progress of the business.

Prepare a price list that is based on solid information. It is always tempting to undersell yourself at the beginning of a new business to attract clients, but this is not a good idea as it will be difficult to raise prices at a later date, and you should charge what you are worth.

Work backwards when setting fees. Put down how much you need to earn to live on for a year, add to that your overheads, including tax, and divide this sum by the number of weeks you are available to work in a year. You now have a weekly amount of income you need to achieve. Divide this again by the amount of hours you will realistically fill with paying clients in a week and this amount will be your hourly treatment charge.

When writing any business plan, be realistic about your statements and look at it regularly. Remember, it is not set in stone and you can adjust it when necessary.

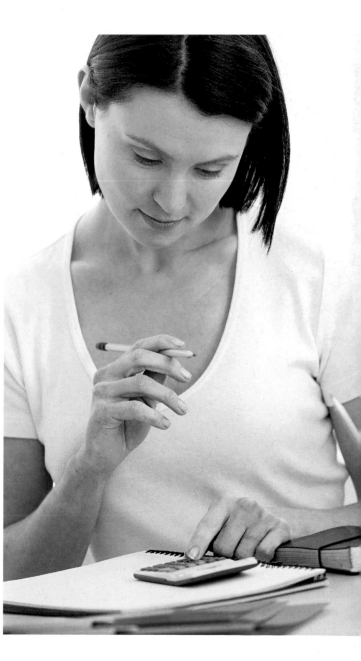

Budgeting Calculate fees based on solid information and review the levels annually, taking into account any changes in your overheads, the market and the economic climate.

Marketing and promotion

Once your massage practice is set up, your next task is to get clients through the door. Although this may seem a daunting task at first, rest assured it will get easier as you build up your client base and word gets around.

Marketing involves promoting your business, its image, what you do and the direction you are going. You will need to identify where your potential clients are and be aware of local competition. Find out what other therapists charge, what their premises are like and what services they offer. Look for opportunities: if your competitor is closed on Thursdays and every day at 6pm, offer promotions on Thursdays and have one night a week where you offer appointments until 7pm.

Many small businesses fail in the first three years, primarily through lack of market research, so it is important to spend time planning and implementing a proper marketing strategy.

The following are simple ideas that will not cost huge amounts of money to carry out.

Literature

Choose an image, name or logo that reflects your style of the business. For instance, if you want to promote a clinical massage service choose a clean, slightly corporate look rather than an eco-natural design of an earthier therapist. If you want to work in a sports environment, choose images associated with athletes and gyms. Make sure that all your literature is consistent, using the same fonts, logos and colours, and that it always contains the most important piece of information clearly: your contact telephone and email details. If working from home, avoid giving out your full address on promotional literature, an area name will suffice.

It is a good idea to design your literature with a dual purpose: business cards can also be appointment cards on the reverse; brochures about your services can also be informative posters.

Once you have business cards, brochures and posters, identify the venues likely to be frequented by potential customers and ask if you can display them there. It may be a local hotel that does not have an in-house therapist or a golf club whose members regularly have massage. Explore your area and you will be amazed at the opportunities that present themselves.

Website

A simple website is relatively easy to design and there are many internet service providers offering a do-it-yourself package of website, email addresses and hosting the site for a very small cost per month. Make sure that your site is revisited on a regular basis by putting up interesting information and perhaps having a 'massage of the month' promotion.

Advertising

Paid advertising is usually very costly and will not necessarily bring in clients immediately. If you cannot afford regular placements to endorse your branding, there is little return from a one-off advertisement unless it is what is known as 'advertorial', an advertisement with a piece of editorial attached. Advertorial pieces can work well if you choose your topic carefully so that it grabs the readers' attention.

Regular press releases sent out to relevant papers and magazines may also result in them printing a piece about your business.

Networking

Networking through local clubs, business network groups or with other therapists can be productive. You could offer to give a talk or demonstration, or offer a special promotion. Other therapists may welcome your assistance as a locum or might be willing to join together in promotional activities.

Joining an association or body will also put you in touch with network groups in your area and add you to their register of approved therapists.

Existing clients

Last but not least, remember to nurture your existing clients, show appreciation for their continuing business by sending them a card on special occasions such as birthdays, holidays and other events. This is a simple tool to make them feel special and remind them you are still around if they have not been to see you for a while. Offer

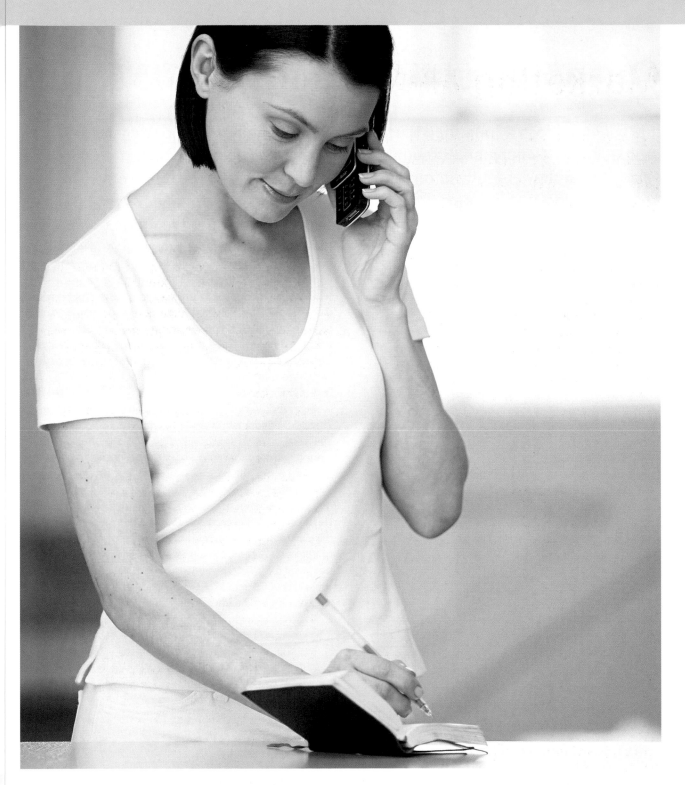

them incentives if they refer a new client or book a block of treatments. Most of all ensure that each massage you give is to the best of your ability and that the client treated in a professional manner, as word of mouth is the best marketing tool and the cheapest.

Promotion You will have to make the effort to promote your business in order to build up your client base. Explore your local area to find opportunities to market your treatments.

Bowen Technique

Developed in Australia by a therapist called Thomas A. Bowen, this system aims to rebalance the body by using gentle moves on the tissues, in particular the fascia. Bowen moves are made at key structural parts in the body that the brain uses to determine posture, so techniques applied at these points will have a profound effect on the way the body holds itself.

A Bowen practitioner intuitively feels where the muscles are tense and uses these moves as a release mechanism.

Chiropractic

A chiropractor works specifically on the spine, manipulating the vertebrae in an effort to relieve pain and release any impingements that are causing discomfort. The principle applied is that pain is generally caused by a nerve

Chiropractic A chiropractor may treat the neck for problems, along with head, shoulders or arms. Treatment consists of adjustments to free joints and reduce spinal nerve irritation.

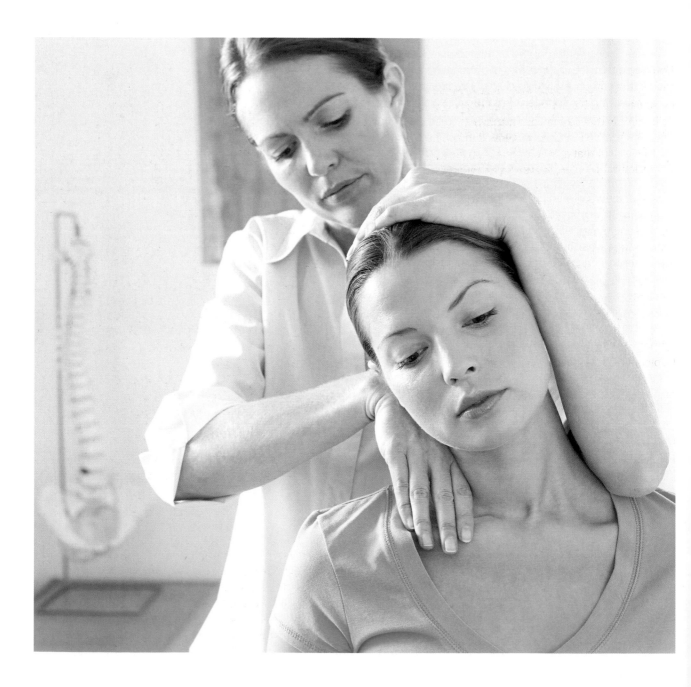

malfunctioning and as the spinal cord houses the central nervous system, it becomes the focus of the treatment.

Chiropractic is often successful in the treatment of neck pain, headaches and lower back pain.

Homeopathy

This is the science of treating like with like. Miniscule doses of the cause of a condition, whether bacteria, virus or other substance, are administered in tablet or liquid form in order to build up the patient's resistance and immunity.

Homeopathic remedies need to be stored and taken away from any strong smells that could impair their effectiveness.

Osteopathy

Unlike a chiropractor, an osteopath manipulates both the muscular and skeletal structures of the body. The basis of their work is that structure and function cannot be treated separately; if the structure sustains damage it will affect the function in that area. Manipulation aims to correct the structural problem and so improve the function.

Physiotherapy

A massage therapist often works alongside a physiotherapist, warming up areas to be treated. A physiotherapist uses exercise and stretching to rehabilitate the body after accident, surgery or illness. Some physiotherapists are also trained in massage and will apply pressure through trigger points to help relieve muscle soreness and tension.

Reflexology

Depicted in drawings on the walls of the ancient tombs in Egypt, this therapy uses the soles of the feet as maps to locate problem areas in the body. There are points or zones of the feet known as reflexes that correspond to organs of the body; for example, the tips of the toes represent the sinuses. Using finger or thumb pressure, the reflexologist works over these points and where a reflex reacts painfully, applies gentle pressure in order to help the corresponding part of the body to heal.

Reiki

A mixture of hands-on therapy and spiritual healing, Reiki means 'universal life force' in Japanese. This discipline has become popular worldwide and there are many accepted forms.

A person practising Reiki is regarded as a healer rather than a therapist, as they act as a channel between the energy and the client. They make contact with their hands

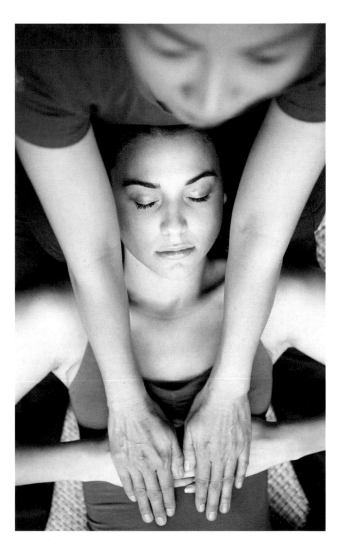

Reiki This relaxing therapy promotes balance through spiritual healing and energy channelling. Once trained in the discipline, you are seen as a healer, rather than a therapist.

on different parts of the client's body, through clothing, and are believed to draw energy into the client's body, promoting relaxation, balance and natural healing.

Shiatsu

A Shiatsu practitioner works on a floor mat, with their client fully clothed and uses pressure points and passive stretching to help relaxation, address specific conditions and promote natural healing. It is a form of acupressure, the practitioner using their finger or thumb pads to apply pressure to specific points along the meridians. A course of treatments is recommended to achieve maximum benefit, the positive after-effects building up week by week.

Acknowledgements

I would like to give special thanks to Jennifer Wayte and John French of the Federation of Holistic Therapists for their kind support, those who kept me on track especially Netty, Marian, Nicki et al, and Jim and Lianne who have shared their inspiring habitat.

Executive editor Jessica Cowie

Editor Ruth Wiseall

Executive art editor Penny Stock

Designer Peter Gerrish

Illustrator Cactus Design and Illustration Ltd

Picture researcher Taura Riley

Production controllers Hannah Burke and Linda Parry

Special photography © Octopus Publishing Group Ltd/Russell Sadur

Other photography
Alamy/Bubbles Photography 44; Chris Rout 48; Martin Lee 56.
Bridgeman Art Library 11; © ADAGP, Paris and DACS, London 2008 13.
Corbis UK Ltd/Emely/zefa 249; Image Source 30.
Getty Images/Alex Mares-Manton 17.
Jupiterimages/Matthew Wakem 28; Pedro Del Rio 61.
Mary Evans Picture Library/Lionel Coates 12.
Masterfile/Andy Lee 68.
Octopus Publishing Group Limited/Russell Sadur 20, 190; Ruth Jenkinson 246.
Punchstock/Digital Vision 92.
Royalty-Free Images/PhotoDisc 247; Photolibrary 26.
Science Photo Library/Adam Gault 248; Coneyl Jay 47.
Shutterstock/jkitan 15.